NOURISHED BY FAITH

NOURISHED
BY FAITH

Biblical Perspective on Food, Eating Disorders, and Body Image

ANNA MARIE LONG MS, RD, LD, CEDS-C
& STEPHANIE BROWN

TABLE OF CONTENTS

PREFACE

"May the God of hope fill you with all joy and peace in believing, so that by the power of the Holy Spirit you may abound in hope."

- Romans 15:13 (ESV)

WE ARE SO glad you found this book. If you are coming from a place of curiosity and have never heard the term "diet culture" before, welcome. If you are familiar with disordered eating patterns and this is not new information, this book is for you, too. If you have never heard of the term diet culture, it is probably because diets and disordered eating are normalized in our society, so you have never noticed or thought otherwise. Diet culture is a cultural force that prioritizes and emphasizes thinness, appearance, and shape over true health. Diet culture pushes misinformation about food by labeling it as "good" and "bad." It is found in the awful language people use against their bodies and other's bodies. It is in the constant editing of pictures and videos and feelings of needing to restrict food or compensate with exercise for some appearance-based goal or health myth. "Healthism" (the idea that you are the one completely in control of your health and appearance) can also be a consequence of diet culture. This belief is far from the truth. Our book aims to describe the ways diet culture deceives us and has even found its way into the church. While diet culture claims "health," it instead has led to a vast number of people struggling with disordered eating, mental health, and negative body image, whether visibly or invisibly. After all, what does a healthy relationship between food and body image look like?

Body image has been a topic that continues to gain attention. Most people cannot go a week, let alone a few days, without hearing someone comment on their own body or someone else's body. You cannot scroll on social media, drive down a highway, or watch TV and movies without seeing bodies in your face. You cannot listen to music without someone's body being mentioned in it. Not to mention, the bodies you see are often all different. Sometimes, it is the stick-thin body, then it is the toned body or bulked body, and then it is the thick body. People commonly give terms to stereotype bodies; "the model body," the "slim thick," the "gym-bro," the "dad bod", etc. Nonetheless, the "ideal body" is forever changing while the noise around bodies ever increases. Throw in diet industry marketing, conflicting health research, blog posts, med-spas left and right, influencer "tips and tricks," and misinformed doctors on nutrition; it is no wonder there is so much confusion around what we should do with our bodies.

Disordered eating involves creating labels and categories for food, restricting intake, compulsive intake, rigid eating patterns, and chronic dieting, as a few examples. Disordered eating is usually a precursor to an eating disorder. Eating disorders can be defined by the Diagnostic and Statistical Manual, 5th edition (DSM-V). However, people who do not fit into diagnostic boxes struggle every day. A simple Google search can give you diagnostic information as defined by the DSM-V, but at the end of the day, the diagnosis may or may not describe someone perfectly. Often, health insurance dictates coverage for eating disorder care. Not having a "textbook diagnosis" denies thousands of people the care they need. The reality is that disordered eating is all too common, and using diagnostic criteria to validate or invalidate your struggles is not helpful. If you think you may have an eating disorder (whether or not you fit all or no diagnostic criteria), seek help from an eating disorder specialist, registered dietitian, therapist, or doctor.

The reality is, nutrition is highly individualized. As much as you may be hoping this book would be yet another "solution" to what you are wanting, it is not. There is no black-and-white "solution." Rather, the true solution to body image struggles is finding contentment outside of the appearance of your body. Contentment is not a place you reach once; rather, it is an active pursuit. The source of true contentment lies in our perfect Creator. This book will, indeed, point you to the Truth, and provide you with rhetorical questions, facts, and practical steps toward freedom, but we fully believe that apart from the Spirit of God, nothing can happen. God is the only one who can provide you with true and lasting contentment, and we hope this book points you to Him. The most important thing we hope you get from this book is that your relationship with God must be primary; everything else is secondary. This includes your relationship with food and your body! If you do not have a firm foundation on Christ, the one who never fails, placing your foundation on your body surely will fail. If you do not know Jesus as your Lord and Savior, this book is also for you. This book explains what Jesus has done for us and how Jesus can meet you. It is our hope and prayer that in reading this book, you will come to know Christ, and He will meet you in your struggles, and that ultimately (and more importantly), this will lead you to a saving faith.

While the Bible never explicitly uses the term eating disorders or disordered eating, it does speak a great deal about our bodies and food. God's Word is living and active (Hebrews 4:12), so principles can be derived from Truth to apply to situations like disordered eating and eating disorders (similar to how dating is not Biblical yet has Biblically-derived principles). Though our book does aim to provide a Biblical perspective, some things in this book are opinion/professional views on the subject based on our experience. The reality is you can find countless resources out there on the topic of food and body image. Technology allows us endless access to books, blogs, documentaries, and podcasts. You can even find many Christian-equipping resources on the topic of body image! However, as we have read various resources, we have realized in general, there are wonderful books on body image theologically and wonderful books scientifically, but rarely are there books that are both theologically-sound and scientifically based on evidence and clinical experience.

Filling this gap is the goal of our book! In the book, you will notice scripture incorporated throughout. That is because we want you to know what the Word of God says, not what we say. Our goal is to take the pieces of scripture that "self-help" books have misused and do our best to refocus our eyes back on God and the authorial intent of each passage or piece of scripture included. This book will hopefully help you tackle some scripture, especially those verses and passages commonly taken out of context in attempts to justify diet culture beliefs. While this book's approach is practical theology, we do not want to see theology from man's perspective, whether that be the lens of diet culture or even the lens of weight-neutral healthcare reading it. It is dangerous to try to put God into a box of your niche interest. We need to understand our perspective as God's creatures here on earth with purpose.

Our number one prayer in this book is that you realize the gospel is essential. Man was made in the image of God, yet because of sin, we fell. Christ came in full deity and humanity to pay for our sins. He had a bodily resurrection, and we are thus saved by faith alone through grace alone, and Jesus will return. With this as the foundation, this book will constantly point you to the gospel of Jesus Christ, but this book also is written from Biblically-derived and Spirit-empowered convictions. Thus, some of the information we present in this book you may disagree with, and that is okay! After all, the only book that is perfectly pure and without fault is the Bible. Our goal is not to change your mind or project our beliefs onto you, but it is to faithfully steward our passions, research, and the Word of God to those who will read. Convictions are secondary and can differ, but we can agree to disagree to promote unity within the body of believers rather than the disunity the enemy desires. We do pray the Holy Spirit will do something powerful in your heart and life through this book.

As mentioned, throughout this book there will be scripture references and references to other books and relevant research. We encourage you to study the scriptures provided on your own, too, and ask God to guide your convictions and to find enjoyment in His Word. Use the other citations as resources to continue learning and growing! You can also use this book to have discussions in the context of your community. Take note of what stands out to you or challenges you. Let us begin to normalize talking about these things honestly in church circles. Though many body image resources are unfortunately written solely for women, we realize body image is a topic that heavily affects *both* men and women. Therefore, we have tailored the writing of this book to apply to both. After all, the Lord shows no partiality.

Additionally, while this book will be relevant to those who struggle with body image or their relationship with food, this book is also wonderful for those who have friends and family who struggle or those who want to become more aware and equipped around this idea in our culture. This book is written completely free of diet culture. We also have tried to the best of our ability to be sensitive to any triggers and address those. Therefore, this book is also good for anyone going through eating disorder recovery at any stage of their journey. Lastly, this is a great resource for professionals, both those who are believers in Christ and those who may work with believers and want to become more aware of their clients' worldview and thus, perspective.

Our final disclaimer before we begin is that everyone's story is different, so please do not compare yours to someone else. Some people may be able to read a book like this, find Jesus, and be free from body image struggles. And let us be clear: this book will NOT rescue you from body image struggles; the rescue power lies in Jesus' transforming work on the cross. Others may come to this book 10-15 years into body image struggles and still struggle. The goal is not sobriety of your struggle but total surrender and devotion to worshiping Jesus in all areas of your life, even through the areas that challenge you.

INTRODUCTION

About Anna Marie Long

I GREW UP in a relatively diet-free household. No one in my family made negative comments about food or body, despite my dad working in healthcare. I started taking dance lessons as a young child and eventually fell in love with competitive cheerleading. I did competitive cheer for all of middle and high school, as well as the first two years of college. Cheer and dance are breeding grounds for eating disorders, although I did not think much of the food and body talk that was all around me until late high school and early college.

In my senior year of high school, I decided I wanted to try out for the University of Texas at Austin all-girl cheerleading team. I practiced every day, working on my tumbling skills. The week before the tryout, I felt intense anxiety. My mom could tell that I was feeling anxious, and she reminded me of Philippians 4:6-7, which says, *"Do not be anxious about anything, but in everything by prayer and supplication with thanksgiving let your requests be made known to*

God. And the peace of God, which surpasses all understanding, will guard your hearts and your minds in Christ Jesus." I was not sure what else to do, so I prayed this verse back to God. I told Him about my anxiety, and it felt as if a literal weight was lifted off my shoulders. This was the first time I felt the Holy Spirit move in my life. I wish I could say my life was forever changed after that, but God had a lot more to teach me throughout and after college. One thing was different; I was no longer anxious about the cheer tryout. I went to Austin and tried out for the team. I did not end up making the team, but I felt at peace with this. I was not ready to be finished with cheer, so I tried out and joined a competitive cheer team at a local gym in Austin.

In my freshman year of college, making friends was harder than I anticipated as an extrovert, and my roommate ended up not being the friend I was hoping for. Moving from a small town to a big city with no local community was a difficult transition. In my freshman year, I started going to the gym consistently for the first time and engaging in disordered eating behaviors. I switched my major to nutrition in my sophomore year of college because I was *obsessed* with food. My disordered eating thoughts and behaviors fueled my choice of career path. As a nutrition major, we spent one day in a 3-credit hour lecture learning about eating disorders (the fact that this is all I learned in undergrad still blows my mind). I convinced myself that my disordered thoughts and behaviors were "fine" and I was just "prioritizing my health." I believed the lie from diet culture that if you do not check all the boxes of an eating disorder diagnosis, you are normal.

As college continued, the Lord placed some amazing people in my life who showed me what it looked like to follow Him and trust in Him. I knew that God was good, but my sinful desires led me to live a life that was focused on myself and my body. College and the first few years after were a rollercoaster. God continually showed me more of Himself, but I continued in my own selfishness. I learned about intuitive eating the summer before my senior year of college through a student internship that I had with a local sports dietitian. As I learned more about nutrition and what our bodies need (not just what diet culture says), I began to reintroduce foods that I was restricting. I read the entire intuitive eating book in less than a week and decided that I wanted to be an intuitive eater. Of course, it was not that simple. During my dietetic internship, I was learning and unlearning all of the weight-focused nutrition therapy information I learned in school and relearning how to take a more compassionate, behavior-focused, and client-centered approach. As I was nearing the end of my dietetic internship, I had the opportunity to work with eating disorders in the outpatient setting, and everything just clicked into place. I realized the Lord was calling me to work with eating disorders, to challenge myself to *actually* eat intuitively, and to focus more on Him and less on perfectionism around eating and my body.

For several months before I began working with eating disorders, the Lord was taking away everything that I was finding my identity in and showing me that He was all I needed. The Lord met me where I was and showed me that all I needed to do was abide in Him and trust Him. As I walked with Him and as I transitioned from college student to working professional, my food and body struggles drastically improved. I learned the hard way how not to find my worth and value in my work. I got a job working at an outpatient group practice of therapists specializing in eating disorders. I was the first dietitian to work at the practice, and I loved walking alongside my clients in eating disorder recovery. I learned so much working closely with gifted therapists and will forever be grateful for my time at the group practice.

In 2020, I met my now husband, and we took a theology class together at our church. Through this class, I was able to see that the Bible is not silent on any issue. Scripture actually has a lot to say about the way we view food and our bodies. Once I took this class, I could not "un-see" this and began to talk with friends and colleagues about how the Bible actually speaks to every issue that we face. Compartmentalizing our relationship with food/body as separate from our relationship with Jesus does us a disservice and keeps us stuck.

I married my best friend in 2021. My husband loves the Lord more than anyone or anything, and he constantly points me back to Jesus. I am blessed to have such an encouraging presence by my side. In 2022, he supported my desire to move into private practice and has been my biggest cheerleader ever since. A major reason I moved into private practice was so that I could be more explicit with my marketing around incorporating Christian faith into my work.

In discussing faith with some of my clients, I realized that the Christian clients I worked with truly gave me joy. I felt like our work was making a difference in their lives that would last. Burnout is common in working with eating disorders, but as I was able to talk about how our food and body struggles relate to our relationship with Jesus and what He teaches, I got excited about my work all over again. I have also worked with clients who are non-believers and are questioning their faith. While it is outside of my scope of practice as a dietitian to share my personal faith with them, I have been able to offer the unique perspective of someone who loves scripture and wants others to know and love Jesus too. While my work is not vocational ministry, this is where the Lord has me, and I love getting to support my clients in letting the Lord into their recovery journey every day.

About Stephanie Brown

I GREW UP in a pretty diet-culture-heavy household. I remember weight loss methods being commonplace and watching family members engage in disordered behaviors every day, though never defined as "disordered eating behaviors." I thought these were normal, so I began to engage in my own disordered eating behaviors.

By the time middle school started, I joined a competitive cheer team. As a cheerleader, I vividly remember idolizing the role of a flyer (the one on top of the stunts in cheerleading). During 7th grade competitive cheerleading, I decided to try out for flyer, but my cheer coach did not take me seriously and just laughed at me for my effort. I was instantly angry at my body. That same year, I also got taken out for two months after developing a bulging disk in my lower back. Old comments I had received growing up around my body haunted me, and I convinced myself the reason for my back injury was that I was "too fat." I was always self-conscious about my body during practice. I got bullied for my appearance when I hit puberty and started getting curves before others. I remember getting called a "gorilla" when I started to grow armpit hair and a "pepperoni face" when I developed acne. This made me internalize there was more wrong with my body than just my shape.

During the same time, my mom was diagnosed with breast cancer for the first time. It was quite a shock to my family! By God's grace, she recovered, but a few years later, this cancer returned, and I was stunned. Out of sincere love for my mom, I began to do online "research" through blogs and Google on how this cancer came to be (thus being fed with the endless stream of misinformation on the internet). Because of this, I quickly labeled foods in my head as "good and bad," and was able to "justify" these labels based on the reality of chronic disease existing in my family.

Also, starting in middle school, I bonded with my mom over watching the Bachelor and Bachelorette, which both glamorize unhealthy relationships. This led to me having unrealistic expectations of what "true love is," conclusions that gossip is a way to fend for yourself, and assumptions that you must look 100% put together all the time for men to be attracted to you. This caused me to daydream about high school. I had it in my mind that once high school started, it would be a new beginning for me: "New school, new year, new me."

This construct in my mind, as well as the development of an obsession with "healthy foods," led me to a destructive cycle of undereating and overexercising. Lots of life circumstances at the time were out of my control (a natural disaster, parental marital struggles, and my brother moving out for college), so food easily became a control mechanism and exercise a distraction. I had all the classic symptoms of a life-threatening eating disorder, yet I did not see anything wrong with myself. When I hit rock bottom during my freshman year of high school, my cheer coach asked me if I was eating enough. She introduced me to what an eating disorder was, and low and behold, a few months later, I found myself diagnosed with Anorexia Nervosa (as well as other mental health diagnoses) and started meeting with an eating disorder therapist.

After many appointments, therapy sessions, and several long years later, I slowly began to restore weight. In cheerleading, I broke my nose twice within the span of three months and was forced to sit out of my activities to heal. Though I was angry at the time, I now believe in retrospect that the Lord, in His kindness, allowed this to happen, knowing that if left to myself, I would have continued in this destructive cycle of over-exercising.

In my junior year of high school, I met a girl in one of my classes who invited me to her birthday party. Here, I realized all her friends were from a church group, and I joined their Bible study. We studied the book of Ecclesiastes, and I remember being so blown away by how relevant the Bible was to me in my life at that time. Though I did not let these girls into what was going on in my life then, I knew I wanted to stay around them, so I started attending church with them when I could. My prior view of the church had been just a religious concept. It was boring to me, and I was uninterested. The groups I had tried always felt like social hours more than anything life-changing, and I never understood how God and Jesus related. I believed the lie that I would never understand anything since I did not grow up in the church.

COVID-19 hit at the end of my junior year, and I was isolated again. With a sudden increase in free time, I began to watch church sermons broadcast online. My curiosity about Jesus continued to grow. With gyms closed and cheer practice canceled, I was further forced out of excessive exercise. I did not see my peers as often, so comparisons became less forefront of my mind. It was during this time I was able to really practice intuitive eating. I could eat what I wanted when I wanted and didn't have to worry about packing lunches or getting hungry in class.

During my senior year, I had the choice to remain virtual or go back in person, and I chose to remain virtual. Getting to focus on my mental health and pursuit of Jesus that year was one of the most crucial times of my life. However, this did not mean there wasn't a struggle. I began to pray for a Christ-centered community in college, and low and behold, the summer going into my freshman year, I met another group of girls. We read through the Gospel of John. They showed me what it looked like to have a quiet time and how to pray through Scripture. I also heard their testimonies and remember thinking to myself, "If God can do that in their lives, what could he do in mine?" I wrestled with the fact that I had apparent success in my life without Jesus, but it hit me that I was living only for myself. So it was during that season that I decided to fully surrender to Jesus and center my entire life around Him before starting college. Because of this, I felt such peace coming into college, and I can undoubtedly say the Lord has moved in and through my life in ways in which I could never have imagined for myself (and that makes me super excited for the future). I chose to major in nutrition, though I did not know the exact route I wanted to take with it. I became super fascinated with all the myths that were debunked and the behavioral research that was involved. I also took part in a gospel recovery program at my church. With these passions growing, I began to pray for opportunities that could incorporate gospel-centered recovery into those struggling with eating disorders. I wanted to be able to incorporate both science-backed, evidenced-based eating disorder research and information along with theologically sound and scripturally backed truths, as well as my own story. Then, I met Anna Marie through my local church, and she graciously asked me if I wanted to intern with her. This has been an incredible gift in my life.

When I thought back to my eating disorder recovery, it was a clear sign of the Lord pursuing me before I was ever pursuing Him. Through interning with Anna Marie and my local church, my eyes were opened to my deep love for soul care. With this love, I am now pursuing a Master of Human Services Counseling and a recovery ministry residency before I complete my dietetic rotations to become a Registered Dietitian. I am also a Certified Personal Trainer and group fitness instructor, and I strive to help people move their bodies in a way that feels good and joyful to them.

When I think back to my expectations going into college versus where the Lord brought me at the end of college, it is radically different. He has proven to be my portion every single day. He gives us what we can handle and when we can handle it. Ever since committing my life to Jesus, He has drastically reformed my view of body image, work and rest, school, community, dating relationships, and marriage.

I went into college, like high school, daydreaming about all the date events, semi-formals, and formals. I was ashamed that I had never been asked to homecoming or prom or asked on a single date in high school. But God has defined his relationship with me over and over again, and that is enough. Even when I am not confident in myself, He makes me secure. I know that my singleness has nothing to do with my body. I do not have to wait it out and play games for men to decide I am good enough. I lack nothing because Jesus has been in total pursuit of my life from before the foundation of the world. No relationship status, number of friends, grade, financial amount, weight on a scale, or number of Instagram likes could ever take my identity away from, first and foremost, being a daughter of God. This identity is the fuel through which everything else from my life now flows. Christ reigns at the center. Loving people, despite how they make me feel or what they give me in return, is now an opportunity I have to demonstrate the spiritual reality of Jesus' love for me. At the end of the day, the biggest, truest, most life-changing thing about me is God's selfless, sacrificial, and dignity-driven love.

1

IMAGE OF GOD

"Then God said, 'Let us make man in our image, after our likeness. And let them have dominion over the fish of the sea and over the birds of the heavens and over the livestock and over all the earth and over every creeping thing that creeps on the earth.' So God created man in his own image; in the image of God, he created him; male and female, he created them. And God blessed them. And God said to them, 'Be fruitful and multiply and fill the earth and subdue it, and have dominion over the fish of the sea and over the birds of the heavens and over every living thing that moves on the earth.'"
~ Genesis 1:26-28 (ESV)

GOD CARES ABOUT food, and He cares about your relationship with your body. To gain a deeper understanding of why God cares, it is necessary to study what it means to be created in the image of God. In secular and religious circles alike, "What is the meaning of life?" is a common question. While one might find various answers to these questions on a bookshelf or on Google, scripture makes the answer abundantly clear: we were created by God to glorify God. Humans are broken, imperfect pictures of our perfect, all-powerful Creator. Regardless of body shape, shade, or size, we have value.

Our bodies are not merely shells to house our souls, but our physical bodies have inherent value along with our hearts, minds, and souls.[1] Looking back to the creation of man, Genesis 2:7 says, *"the Lord God formed the man of dust from the ground and breathed into his nostrils the breath of life."* Notice how God actually *formed* our physical body before he breathed life into it. [1] This forming of our physical body broke the rhythm of the rest of creation. In other words, we see distinction in our forming because, throughout Genesis 1, we are told that God *spoke* the earth into existence. God said, *"Let there be..."* and there was!

Moreover, God sees so much value in physical bodies that He gave one to Himself in Jesus Christ! Jesus came fully in bodily flesh yet remained fully God! Colossians 2:9 expresses this dual nature of Jesus, stating, *"the whole fullness of deity dwells bodily"* (Colossians 2:9).

Isaiah 43:7 also tells us that God formed us, and He called us to reflect His glory. Glory is defined as "praise, honor, or distinction" and "worshipful praise, honor, and thanksgiving."[2] Therefore, we glorify God by worshiping, beautifying, and obeying Him. We magnify His name. We do not magnify our own name by the way we look or "manage" our bodies. Our natural inclination is toward self-centeredness, but our purpose as humans is to enjoy God forever (John 10:10, Psalm 16:11). As image bearers, we reflect God's character and purposes in our humanity.

We are meant to be an image of our Creator. Let us use an illustration to see what it is like to be made in God's image. While it is important to note that every example will fall short of truly reflecting God's glory, illustrations are helpful nonetheless. Imagine you are the parent of a four-year-old son. Your family has plans to go to Disney World. Leading up to the trip, you tell your child all about Disney and how he will get to "experience the magic" and meet Mickey Mouse. You show him pictures of your past trips to Disney. The more your child learns about Disney World, the more excited he is to go. He begins to ask, "How many more days?" and "Can you show me the pictures again?" The more he anticipates what to expect, the more excited he gets. However, in all of your pictures, the castle does not look as magical as you remember in person. While the pictures can be helpful to excite your 4-year-old son, they will not compare to when he is there experiencing the magic himself. While this is an imperfect example (God is *so much* greater than Disney World), we are the pictures, and God is the real experience. The more we learn about who God is and see Him reflected in other believers, the more excited we get to spend eternity with Him. As we understand God more and grow in intimacy with Him, we can recognize and understand the true meaning and bigger purpose in this life.

Our purpose is not to micromanage the bodies God has given us as vessels to reflect Himself. When we endlessly pursue changing our bodies, we are deviating from God's design. Our society, or diet culture, constantly sends us messages contrary to this truth. Diet culture refers to the pervasive messaging that places extreme value on body size, muscle mass, and thinness. Our culture has become obsessed with yo-yo dieting (losing weight and regaining it) in attempts to reach an unrealistic ideal.

Psalm 139:13 says that *"God knitted [us] together in [our] mother's womb,"* then we are called *"fearfully and wonderfully made"* (Psalm 139:14). The Western idea of body mass index (BMI) as an indicator of health status contradicts God's perfect design for true health. Diet culture perpetuates the "thin ideal" that claims smaller bodies are superior and that thinness is synonymous with health. Nowhere in scripture does it say that smaller bodies, or any other societally praised bodies, are more in the image of God than bodies that do not live up to the "thin ideal."

If you are spending hours at the gym or on Pinterest finding "healthy recipes," this may be a sign that "health" or being at a smaller weight has become an object of your worship. **Your attention determines your devotion.** We must ask ourselves: are we worshiping the One True God, or are we worshiping ourselves? In what ways are we gratifying our flesh instead of what Jesus wants for our bodies? Are we walking in slavery to diet culture or freedom in Christ? Colossians 1:15-16 says, *"[Jesus] is the image of the invisible God, the firstborn of all creation. For by him, all things were created, in heaven and on earth, visible and invisible, whether thrones or dominions or rulers or authorities—all things were created through him and for him."* He is our Creator, and the God of reconciliation. Sin disrupts our relationship with God, ourselves, one another, and creation, yet Jesus has made a way for us to be restored to a holy God. And He has made a way for us to restore our broken relationship with our bodies. We are commanded to eat and drink for the glory of God (1 Corinthians 10:31). As we let Jesus restore our relationship with food and our bodies, we can walk in freedom and learn what it looks like to glorify God even in our eating and drinking.

Once you place your faith and trust in Jesus Christ as your Lord and Savior, you are in Christ, and Christ is in you. If you are in Christ, you have obtained an inheritance (Ephesians 1:11). Ephesians 1:11-14 talks about this inheritance from the moment we first believe and accept Christ as our Savior. This inheritance is getting to spend eternity with your Creator, enjoying Him and His glory forever. Additionally, Romans 8:29 says that *"those whom he foreknew he also predestined to be conformed to the image of his Son."* He has chosen you and adopted you into His family out of His great love. This is the greatest gift we can receive, and it is not dependent on our body size, shape, or "health status." We are His, and we are set free: *"For freedom, Christ has set us free; stand firm therefore, and do not submit again to a yoke of slavery"* (Galatians 5:1). The persistent pursuit of changing your body to be someone you are not becomes a yoke of slavery. Christ has set you free from this. God created your body intentionally and with purpose. In 2 Corinthians 4:4-6, we learn that being created in the image of God lets light shine out of darkness. Satan is the real enemy of God. Satan's work is to blind this light by convincing us God is not good to us and that there is something wrong with us, but God's work of being the light is greater (John 1:5).

. . .

PRAYER

Dear God,

Thank you for creating me in Your image. You are a gracious, loving Father who chose me to bear your likeness. I confess that I can forget the importance of being created to reflect You. I can get caught up in the world and our culture's definitions of attractiveness and health. I have value because I am Your child, and You created me. You do not have the same standards as the world. Help me to align my view of myself with the way that You view me as an image-bearer. Show me what it looks like to walk in freedom and glorify You in the way that I eat, drink, and treat my body.

In Jesus' name, amen.

SOURCES:

1. Allberry S. *What God Has to Say about Our Bodies: How the Gospel Is Good News for Our Physical Selves*. Wheaton, Illinois: Crossway; 2021.
2. "Glory." Merriam-Webster.com Dictionary, Merriam-Webster, https://www.merriam-webster.com/dictionary/glory. Accessed 12 Jan. 2023.

2

WORLDLY STANDARDS

OF HEALTH

Defining Body Mass Index (BMI)

"I praise you, for I am fearfully and wonderfully made.
Wonderful are your works; my soul knows it very well."
Psalm 139:14 (ESV)

WHILE THE BIBLE does not discuss body mass index (BMI), it does

discuss food and our bodies in depth. Because our healthcare system

places a strong emphasis on BMI, it is important to understand where

this comes from, as well as how it relates to what God says about our

bodies. As healthcare professionals, our aim is to give information that will hopefully inform the way you interpret current health recommendations. While this chapter is mostly rooted in research, some of the content is conclusions that we, as healthcare providers, have drawn. If you disagree with our professional opinions or would like to do more research on your own, we encourage you to first be prayerful about this pursuit. Aim to see the data through the lens of scripture and what the inerrant Word of God has to say about your body first.

Our medical system commonly uses BMI as an indicator of health status, often equating people in smaller bodies with the epitome of "health" and people in larger bodies as "lazy," "undisciplined," and ultimately "unhealthy." BMI, however, was never meant to measure health status. BMI was invented in the early 1800s by a Belgian man named Adolphe Quetelet. While Quetelet was a mathematician, astronomer, statistician, and sociologist, he was *not* a physician. In fact, while he was a highly academic individual, none of his studies were in the medical field, and he never studied medicine. His BMI studies aimed to create a bell curve to define the "average man" of Belgian and Dutch descent.[1] As a statistician, Quetelet was observing trends in populations, not individuals. This bell curve was never intended to describe Americans, Africans, Asians, or any other race/ethnicity that is not Belgian or Dutch. It also was never meant to describe women! Yet, it is used today in an attempt to define the health status of all Americans.

BMI is calculated by weight in kilograms divided by height in square meters. If you are a math person, you may be thinking that a height in meters squared does not make sense. Weight divided by height did not create the normal distribution Quetelet was looking for, but height-squared did. Regardless, BMI only takes height and weight into account and has no actual indicators of internal health. What this means is it does not take muscle mass, frame size, or body composition into account.

In the early 1900s, the World Health Organization (WHO) began using BMI as an indicator of health status due to the observation that an "average" BMI was correlated with longer life expectancy.[1] However, any basic statistics class will teach that correlation does not equal causation. The only two data points taken into account were height and weight, when in reality, social determinants of health, such as socioeconomic status, neighborhood/built environment, access to healthcare, and others, have a larger impact on life expectancy than body size.[2] The Centers for Disease Control and Prevention (CDC) began to place BMI into pathologizing categories such as "overweight" and "obese." Because the terms "overweight" and "obese" can be difficult for some individuals, and because of the stigma associated with them, we will be using quotes. These terms are used here to refer to the medical terms that people are familiar with, even though we strongly disagree with these categories and how the cutoffs are determined. Our current healthcare system and diet culture perpetuates the idea that if we don't micromanage our bodies, we will end up in the dreaded "obese" category, a category that was never defined by the original inventor of the BMI.

Interestingly, in 1995, the National Institutes of Health (NIH) in the United States classified people with a BMI of 27.8 or greater for men and 27.3 or greater for women as being "overweight," based on statistical data from the National Health and Nutrition Examination Study (NHANES) II.[1] In 1998, the cutoff for "overweight" was decreased to 25 for both men and women, based on a decision of 9 medical experts chosen by the NIH (8 of which had financial ties to the weight loss industry). A consequence of this decision was that at least 50% of Americans were now classified as "overweight" or "obese".[1] A significant number of Americans went from being a "normal weight" (BMI between 25-27) to being "overweight" overnight with no changes to their bodies! This is not how God designed us to view our bodies. This continues the wrong belief that God made mistakes when he created us, which could not be further from the truth!

To be clear, classifying individuals as "overweight" or "obese," according to our current medical definitions, only takes into account height and weight and no other factors. Contrary to popular belief, someone who is diagnosed as "overweight" or "obese" may not have any other health risk factors. Our society and medical system rely on the belief that having a BMI that is above "normal" *causes* diseases, such as diabetes, cardiovascular disease, high cholesterol, cancer, etc. However, while a higher weight can be *correlated* with these conditions, there is no evidence to prove that weight itself (independent of health behaviors) *causes* any adverse health outcomes. Two things can be correlated without having a causal relationship. For example, ice cream sales and violent crime rates are very closely correlated.[3] This does not mean that selling more ice cream *causes* more violent crimes. There are always confounding variables.

A peer-reviewed study published in 2016 found that classifying someone's health status based solely on BMI leads to the misclassification of an estimated 74 million US adults![4] This study aimed to compare individuals' health status based solely on BMI with health status based on cardiometabolic markers. Looking at the data based on BMI, anyone with a BMI >25 was classified as "unhealthy." The researchers then observed the lab data and classified anyone with elevated or abnormal blood pressure, triglycerides, cholesterol, or glucose labs as "unhealthy." When the data was compared, the results were shocking. Nearly half of the individuals who were "overweight" based on BMI were cardio-metabolically healthy, and 29% of the individuals who were "obese" were cardio-metabolically healthy. For those at a "healthy" weight based on BMI, 30% of individuals were cardio-metabolically unhealthy.[4] This data shows that health status is much more than weight status and that someone's mere size does not tell us anything about their true physical health.

If you are thinking, "my doctor told me to lose weight to improve my health," you are not alone. The purpose of presenting this information is not to discourage you from the desire to achieve optimal physical health. Actually, it is the opposite. By presenting weight loss as the main way (or only way) to improve health status, medical professionals do many individuals a major disservice. Physical health is multifaceted. You may have heard, "you need to lose weight to manage or prevent diabetes" (or any other physical health concern). While the intention here can be helpful, this does not focus on behavior change and what is actually within someone's control.

Making dietary or lifestyle changes can absolutely be helpful in the management and prevention of chronic diseases. However, advising someone to lose weight without giving them practical tools ultimately makes the goal the wrong thing (i.e., the goal is weight change, not behavior change). Someone could make changes to their lifestyle and lose weight but still have no clue how to manage their blood glucose levels. On the other hand, someone else could learn ways to manage their blood sugar and not lose weight, but they would still achieve the goal of blood sugar management. This individual *may* lose weight, but the point is to place their efforts on the *actual* health issue (management or prevention of diabetes), not on weight. There are behavior changes that anyone can make at any body size to improve their physical health status. Focusing on weight as the main issue only leads to shame and discouragement, and in the end, does not improve health outcomes. Chapter 10 will go into detail on what it looks like to promote health from a dietary perspective without focusing on weight as an outcome or indicator of true health.

The statement that smaller bodies are not more valued by God may be controversial to some because a common thought is, "Well, shouldn't I try to lose weight to be healthy?" As image-bearers, we are, indeed, to steward the bodies that God has given us well. As much as it is within our control, we should strive to live a healthy, balanced lifestyle. However, this idea of body stewardship is very skewed. We will look at this much more throughout the rest of the book. However, as has been discussed, health is not a number on the scale. According to the CDC, health is "a state of physical, mental, and social well-being and not merely the absence of disease and infirmity."[5] Numerous studies show that focusing on weight loss is ineffective at producing thinner, healthier bodies.[6] Rather, focusing on weight as an outcome of health leads to unintended negative consequences, including weight cycling, reduced self-esteem, and eating disorders, among others.[6] Perhaps this is why, despite lowering the BMI cutoff for "normal weight," we have seen an increase in overall average BMI among Americans.[6] On the contrary, we have also seen an increase in life expectancy in Americans over the last several decades.[6] Again, correlation does not equal causation. This increase could be attributed to many factors (such as advancements in medical technology), but it is worth mentioning.

. . .

PRAYER

Dear God,

Thank You for all of the ways that medicine and research have become more advanced over the last few decades. I confess all of the times I have relied on this information instead of trusting in Your perfect design. Help me put research in its place as a helpful tool, but not my savior. Help me to avoid idolizing my health, but at the same time to steward the body that You have given me well.

In Jesus' name, amen.

S O U R C E S :

1. Nuttall, F. Q. Body mass index: Obesity, BMI, and health: A critical review. *Nutrition today.* 2015. https://www.ncbi.nlm.nih.gov/pmc/articles/PMC4890 841/

2. Javed Z, Valero-Elizondo J, Maqsood MH, et al. Social determinants of health and obesity: Findings from a national study of US adults. *Obesity.* 2022;30(2):491-502. doi:https://doi.org/10.1002/oby.23336

3. Bhandari P. Correlation vs. Causation | Difference, Designs & Examples. Scribbr. Published July 12, 2021. https://www.scribbr.com/methodology/correlation-vs-causation/#:~:text=For%20example%2C%20ice%20cre am%20sales

4. Tomiyama AJ, Hunger JM, Nguyen-Cuu J, Wells C. Misclassification of cardiometabolic health when using body mass index categories in NHANES 2005–2012. *International Journal of Obesity.* 2016;40(5):883-886. doi:https://doi.org/10.1038/ijo.2016.17

5. World Health Organization. Constitution of the World Health Organization. *World Health Organization.* Published 2024. https://www.who.int/about/governance/constitution

6. Bacon, L., Aphramor, L. Weight science: Evaluating the evidence for a paradigm shift. *Nutr J 10*, 9 (2011). https://doi.org/10.1186/1475-2891-10-9

3

KNOWING GOD

How a Relationship with God Impacts Our Health Narrative

"Make me to know your ways, O Lord; teach me your paths. Lead me in your truth and teach me, for you are the God of my salvation; for you, I wait all day long."
~Psalm 25:4-5 (ESV)

WE CAN GLORIFY God because we are made in His image. To fully understand Imago Dei (what it means to be made in the image of our Creator), we must seek to understand who God is and what His character is like. Since we are created in the image of God, it is essential to know the true and only God as He has revealed Himself through His Word.

According to *Systematic Theology: First Edition* by Wayne Grudem, to know God, God must reveal Himself to us (Ephesians 1:17-18).[1] We can never *fully* understand God because we are finite humans, and He is infinite. God certainly reveals Himself to us through His creation, as well as through His Word (the Bible). Ultimately, though, God has revealed Himself to us through His one and only Son, Jesus Christ. Because of the incomprehensibility of God, we will never run out of things to learn about Him, nor will we ever tire of discovering more about Him. As we get to know God, we need scripture to interpret what we learn about God so we can understand His character rightly.[1] Rather than striving to define God using our own terms—and putting ourselves at risk of worshiping a god of our own making— we look to God to reveal Himself to us through His Word. Nothing God reveals about Himself will contradict what is written in the Bible. If you believe that God has revealed something about His character to you, make sure it is consistent with what He has revealed about Himself in scripture. If what you think He has revealed is contradictory to His Word, it is not from God. In fact, it could be from the enemy.

Take, for example, Sarah, a former client of mine. [A] In a season when Sarah was feeling dissatisfied with her body, her discipleship group decided to start fasting once a month together. The group would fast on the first day of the month from morning until dinner. Her group studied the spiritual discipline of fasting (see chapter 12 to learn more about fasting), and they were clear on the purpose of this practice. Sarah, however, was convinced that when she fasted, she heard a "voice" from God praising her for "eating less calories that day." This "voice" told her to "keep going." Sarah would fast from all food for 3-5 full days, weighing herself several times during these days and feeling better about herself because of her changing body. The "voice" continued to praise her. Sarah ended up in my office because her discipleship group was concerned about her fasting and the ways that her body changed. Through our work together, she was able to see that the Bible never actually tells us to fast for "health reasons," and the Bible never promotes body change as a marker for improved health or self-esteem. She was able to see that the "voice" was not God revealing Himself to her, but it was a voice from the enemy. We know that the enemy can be highly deceitful and comes only to steal, kill, and destroy (John 10:10).

God, on the other hand, desires a personal relationship with us. Matthew 11:28-29 says that Jesus is gentle and lowly of heart. His yoke is easy, and His burden is light. A yoke is a harness that attaches two animals together to lighten the load on both of them. When Jesus says that His yoke is light, He is saying that when He walks alongside you, your burdens are lightened because He is taking on your yoke rather than you having to bear it alone. If you are struggling with negative food thoughts or body image, He wants to walk alongside you and lighten your burden. It is not a simple "pray once, and it's all fixed," but rather, it is letting God into your most difficult thoughts day after day. It can be so easy to compartmentalize your relationship with food as separate from your relationship with Jesus. This is a trap that the enemy wants you to fall into! Jesus is our faithful comforter and friend, as well as our Lord and Savior. Jesus is not intimidated by what we see as burdensome; we can bring all our challenging food and body thoughts to Him. Therefore, pray without ceasing (1

Thessalonians 5:17). When you think that He has heard enough, pray again, because He *wants* to be a part of your healing.

Jesus set the perfect example of what it looks like to pray without ceasing. For example, the last recorded story of Jesus before His betrayal by Judas and subsequent arrest in all three synoptic Gospels is the story of Him praying in the Garden of Gethsemane (see Matthew 26:36-46, Mark 14:32-52, Luke 22:39-53). Jesus prayed and pleaded to the Father three times for this cup (crucifixion) to be taken from Him. He then asked for not His will, but the Father's to ultimately be done. Prayer was an active choice, though Jesus knew the answer to His first prayer would be no. He was well-acquainted with the Father's will to save sinners. In submission to the Father's will, Jesus went to Him humbly. Jesus knew His ultimate fate, yet in His final hours on earth, He chose to pray. In praying so fervently, He sweated blood. He turned to the Father, relying on His relationship with Him and showing us the perfect example of what it looks like to pray and submit to the Father's will.

This shows us how much God values us, praying to Him and trusting Him enough to submit to His will for our lives, even in the midst of suffering. Jesus set an example for us to ask for the Father's will to be done. God does not always say "yes" to every prayer we pray, but he does answer every prayer, whether it be on this side of the Kingdom or the next. These answers may not play out how we expect or want, but when we go to Him, He begins to align our hearts with His ultimate purposes. When we spend time praying and laying all of ourselves before the Father, He can begin to redeem even the things that we do not want to pray about. Romans 8:26 reminds us that when we do not know how or what we ought to pray for, the Holy Spirit intercedes for us. The more we draw near to God and conform to His character, the more we can understand ourselves as image-bearers and the implications of this.

Through prayer, God invites us to let Him into our thoughts and desires that He already knows. God is everywhere, and He knows all things (Proverbs 15:3, Isaiah 43:2, Psalm 139:7, Job 34:21, Colossians 1:17, et al.) God knows us better than we know ourselves. In Romans 9, the author, Paul, highlights and emphasizes that God chooses people for Himself, and He has every right to do so. Paul addresses a hypothetical rebuttal, "Is God unjust?" by highlighting God's right as humanity's maker to choose how He will use them (using Pharaoh's hardened heart in Exodus as an example). God is even sovereign over evil people's hearts! God has just as much right to choose some people to be recipients of his blessing and some (such as Pharaoh) for evil that ultimately accomplishes His purposes.

Likewise, a potter has the right to make one pot for honorable use and another for dishonorable use. Romans 9:19-21 reminds us that God is the One who made us. The clay cannot say to the potter, "*Why did you make me this way?*" God made us with intention, and He knows us intimately. Praise God that we do not have the power or authority to create ourselves.

As we reflect God in our humanity, we are called to be imitators of Him in our actions and the way we love others (Ephesians 5:1). God shares several attributes with humanity, including His love. God loves sinful humans (John 3:16), and we are called to love others as He loves us, even in our sins. God also shares his mercy, grace, justice, patience, and kindness with us. The more time we spend with God, the more we are conformed to His character. As we grow away from God (or neglect drawing near to Him), the more sin will show up in our lives. John 15:6 says, *"If anyone does not abide in me, he is thrown away like a branch and withers; and the branches are gathered, thrown into the fire, and burned."* The more we abide in God, the less we abide in our food and body image struggles, which are the thief's deceptions and a product of sin (although they may or may not be sinful themselves).[B]

By spending time with God through prayer, as well as hearing what He says in scripture, you will conform more to His character. God knows us intimately. As He continually reveals Himself to us, we can see the ways that he is ultimately providing for us through Jesus. Hebrews 4:15 reminds us that *"we do not have a high priest who is unable to sympathize with our weaknesses, but one who in every respect has been tempted as we are, yet without sin."*

Even though Jesus did not live in the 21st century, He suffered every temptation that we have ever faced, yet He did not sin. In *Mere Christianity*, author C.S. Lewis describes Jesus as someone who understands temptation more than we do. We only know how strong temptation is when we resist it. Someone who withstands temptation for only a few minutes then gives in and sins does not know how much harder it will be to resist temptation an hour, or even a day later. Because Christ never gave into temptation, he is the only One who utterly understands its fullness.[2] He gets what it is like to be human and have sinful desires. This means the next time you have an intrusive thought about body image, God understands this, and He wants you to come to him with all of your thoughts and struggles. He is big enough, strong enough, and loving enough to handle it, and He is able to guide us in the midst of it all as He makes us more like Jesus!

God as Provider and Father

"Ask, and it will be given to you; seek, and you will find; knock, and it will be opened to you. For everyone who asks receives, and the one who seeks finds, and to the one who knocks, it will be opened. Or which one of you, if his son asks him for bread, will give him a stone? Or if he asks for a fish, will give him a serpent? If you then, who are evil, know how to give good gifts to your children, how much more will your Father who is in heaven give good things to those who ask him!"
~ Matthew 7:7-11 (ESV)

AS WE SEE God's provision for us through Jesus, He does not just want to provide for our physical needs. He also wants to provide for us emotionally, relationally, spiritually, and practically. Good parents strive to, likewise, meet the entirety of their children's needs. However, because we live in a fallen, sinful world and parents are limited human beings, even the best of parents cannot meet these needs for us perfectly. Only our Heavenly Father can perfectly provide for us. James 4:2-3 expands upon the idea that we often do not have what we need or desire because we do not ask. God *wants* his children to pray to Him as a good father would want his children to talk to him. To understand this, take into consideration these two scenarios:

Scenario 1: A dad gets home from a long day at work and asks his kid how his day was. The kid shortly replies, "Hard," and moves on to ask his dad if he can have some money for a new toy. He gets what he wants and then ignores his dad with his new toy. Ouch!

Scenario 2: A dad gets home from a long day at work and asks his kid how his day was. The kid shortly replies, "Hard," but lingers for a little while. He gets to tell his dad what was hard about his day specifically. Later that night, the dad draws near to his son with compassion and asks if he can play a game with him. They play a game together and get to enjoy intimacy in a parent-child relationship.

Obviously, scenario 2 would be ideal because every good parent longs to be involved in their child's life and will do anything for that. But how much more does God do that with us as His beloved children? He already knows everything about you, and He still wants you to talk with him. It is an absolute gift that, because of Jesus, we can be in conversation with the holy God.

In the Lord's Prayer, we are told to ask each day for daily bread, which is a powerful symbol of the Lord's provision in the Old Testament. The bread was a staple in the Jewish diet at the time, and we even see bread (or manna) rain down from heaven in Exodus 16:4 as the Israelites were in the wilderness. God's provision is also highlighted when Moses was exhorting a new generation to be faithful to the covenant of God reminding them, *"The Lord your God has blessed you in all the works of your hands. He knows you are going through this great wilderness. These forty years the Lord your God has been with you. You have lacked nothing"* (Deuteronomy 2:7). Furthermore, even today, we refer to the family member who brings income into the household as the "breadwinner." It is not a mistake that the term "bread" is still a sign of provision. While we can strive to provide for ourselves and our families, God is our ultimate provider as our Heavenly Father. Now, this does not mean that we can idly sit around, twiddling our thumbs, and waiting for things to miraculously show up for us (though they definitely can). Psalm 127:1 warns against this and tells us anything built apart from the Lord is labor in vain. 1 Corinthians 3:10 furthers this concept and shows us what happens if we do try to build upon any foundation other than Christ. The idea of building (a verb), or laying a foundation is active, so we do not just stop working. We do, however, recognize God is sovereign over every person, thing, and event. This means that through any job loss, job promotion, natural disaster, unexpected gift or bonus, free meal, or food inflation, God still remains working on the throne. In fact, the word "house" used in Psalm 127 symbolizes family. God is a part of your family as your provider and Heavenly Father.

Jesus calls God "Father" more than any other term or characteristic attributed to God the Father by Jesus in the Gospels![3] The craving for a father's love is literally woven into the fabric of creation. Every person desires to be loved, accepted, hoped for, championed, and cared for, and this is what God our Father does for us when we receive from Him.[3] Having learned more about Imago Dei in the first chapter and God's characteristics, how can we *reflect* Jesus if we do not first *receive* from the Lord? It is easy for us to receive the Lord's physical blessings, but how often do we fully receive His tender, unceasing love for ourselves? The gospel is all about receiving this love that God has for us when we do not deserve it.

When we receive Jesus' love for us, we realize Jesus' commands for us are for our own good. Following the Lord's prayer in Matthew 6:5-14, the Lord tells us not to be anxious about what you will eat, drink, or your body (more on this later), but ends the chapter with, *"Seek first the kingdom of God and his righteousness, and all these things will be added to you"* (Matthew 6:33). Now what are *all these things*? Some of these things include food, drink, and shelter. Jesus did not always have the security of food, drink, and shelter. The Bible Project (a non-profit organization that creates resources to help people understand the Bible) goes into depth on this idea, explaining:

"Jesus did not embrace anxious ways of protection or accumulation, and he consistently [taught] his followers to do the same. He was banking everything on God's promise and trusting that the way of love is more satisfying, secure, and safe than any other way. Though we can experience God's Kingdom in part now, especially in communities where others are choosing to live like this, we still suffer in ways that invite us to rely increasingly on God's generous character and His promise to unite His Kingdom with our whole world."[4]

For those who have chosen to follow Jesus, self-preservation and protection are no longer necessary. Many times throughout the Bible, when people were sent by God on a journey, God did not ask them to pack a bunch of bags for as long as they would be gone. When we look at Elijah's journey in 1 Kings 19, we see Elijah resting under a tree after a long day. He was feeling tired and weak. At the moment where he felt defeated, *"an angel of the Lord touched him and said to him, 'Arise and eat.' And he looked, and behold, there was at his head a cake baked on hot stones and a jar of water"* (1 Kings 19:5-6). Here is a vivid example of food, drink, and shelter being provided! The angel's command was simple: rise and eat. After Elijah fed his body, it says he *"went in the strength of that food forty days and forty nights to Horeb, the mount of God"* (1 Kings 19:8). Elijah saw his food as a gift from the Lord and knew the importance of fueling his body so that it may be used for the Lord's journey. Food is a gift to us, too. God did not even have to make food taste good, yet even this is a common grace (funny enough, it was a cake that appeared to Elijah in the above account!). He allows us to cook and cultivate different foods for flavor profiles, textures, and tastes as an act of *worship* to Him.

The enemy wants us to continue giving in to disordered eating. When we find ourselves spending countless hours looking at "What I Eat in a Day" videos or workout videos, planning meals, counting calories or macros, stalking people's Instagram (you name it!), our energy is sucked right out of us. What if this time was spent abiding with Jesus and serving Him and His purposes for your life? God will strengthen you for the specific journey He has for you because He loves you. In this love, He provides for us the fullness of joy in inviting us into His great plan (Philippians 4:19, John 5:10-11). Because He has provided love for us, we get to extend this love to others (1 John 4:19). Through being adopted into the family of God and having a relationship with the Almighty One who can do exceedingly more than we ask or imagine (Ephesians 3:20), we can extend this same blessing to those who have never understood the provision of unconditional love.

For those who have been wounded by their own biological family (more in chapter 7), what comfort we find in Psalm 27:10, which states that even if our family forsakes us, the Lord will receive us!

Jesus' wounds are what we look to when we face our own wounds. The Word of God is what shapes our lens of the world and those around us, not our experiences. The Word is living and active and the Holy Spirit indwells within those who have believed, so we can let truth inform our future experiences (Hebrews 4:12). If your family perpetuates food and body shame, extend grace to yourself today. Jesus has extended never-ending grace to you. Our purpose here on earth is so much greater than ourselves.

· · ·

PRAYER

Father God,

What a miracle it is that You would send what is most precious to you, Your very own Son, down to this broken earth for me - a sinner! Thank You Jesus, for allowing me back into a right relationship with my Father in Heaven. I confess that I have tried micromanaging my own ways to righteousness and fall short every time. Help me to receive Your love as the greatest treasure in my life. Align my desires to want more of You than anything this world has to offer. Because You are a Provider, I am able to live in abundance. Because You are a Father, I know I always have someone watching over me. Hallelujah, You have my best interests at heart. Therefore, I choose to trust You again today. I trust You with the foods I put into my body. I trust You with the design in which You have created me, knowing that You have called me good. Help me to rest in these truths day after day, for You are the bread I need to come to each and every morning for renewal.

In Jesus' name, amen.

FOOTNOTES:

A. For the purposes of this book and maintaining confidentiality, the names used in the examples have all been changed.

B. Whether or not dieting and disordered eating are sinful is highly nuanced. In some scenarios, it is clear that sin is present, while in other situations, the eating disorder may be the product of highly complex mental health struggles. Because of the nuance, we go into this in-depth in chapter 4.

SOURCES:

1. Grudem, W. A. *Systematic theology: An introduction to biblical doctrine.* Grand Rapids, Michigan. Zondervan Pub. House; 2000.

2. Lewis, C. S. *Mere Christianity.* Harpercollins Publishers; 1952.

3. Giglio, L. *Seeing God as a perfect father: And seeing you as loved, pursued, and secure.* Thomas Nelson; 2023.

4. BibleProject. What Matthew 6:33 (Seek First the Kingdom of God) Means. https://bibleproject.com/articles/what-matthew-6-33-seek-first-the-kingdom-of-god-means/. June 16, 2023. Accessed January 15, 2024.

4

SIN DEFINED

"For all have sinned and fall short of the glory of God."
~ Romans 3:23 (ESV)

SIN IS DEFINED as "any failure to conform to the moral Law of God in act, attitude, or nature."[1] While sins can be overtly obvious, such as stealing or hurting others, actions such as telling "a little white lie" or getting angry in traffic are also sinful. Even though different sins have different earthly consequences, all sins are deserving of death. Our sins go deeper than the choices we make throughout the day. Even our thoughts can be sinful. Jeremiah 17:9 says, *"The heart is deceitful above all things, and desperately sick, who can understand it?"* As God reveals Himself to us and we begin to understand Him, we will begin to understand the weight of our sins and our desperate need for a Savior. God cannot sin.

Since we are created in God's image after His likeness, we have an innate desire to be more like God. This can be a good thing if it is not taken to the extreme of replacing God with more of ourselves. As believers, we can try to be like God in a healthy way because of the Holy Spirit working in our hearts. Our moral or human nature, however, is bent toward sin and not God. When Adam and Eve sinned in the garden in Genesis 3:5, Satan said to Eve, *"God knows that when you eat of [the fruit], your eyes will be opened, and you will be like God, knowing good and evil."* Satan is the true deceiver, but he was right about one thing: that they would know good and evil. As soon as they ate the fruit, they realized that they were naked and needed to cover up (Genesis 3:7). Before sin entered the world, there was no need or desire to cover nakedness. As infants, this desire is not present. Infants allow parents to change their diapers with no shame. Babies do not have the cognitive ability to understand what nakedness is. As we enter adolescence and understand what it means to be naked, an innate desire is formed to cover ourselves. We are ashamed of parts of our bodies that should be publicly covered. Shame is quite different from a sense of modesty. This shame was not present before sin entered the world. Satan knew that we were created to reflect God. He also knew that Adam and Eve were dependent on God, so he convinced them that they could take the place of God and reign on the throne of their own lives. God was not surprised when Adam and Eve sinned by eating the forbidden fruit, but He was still deeply saddened.

Humans are born evil, and on our own, we will choose our sin over God every time. Not even one person can do good apart from God (Psalm 14:3). Adam and Eve became aware of their own evil and knew that apart from God, there was nothing good about them (Romans

3:10-12, Romans 7:18). Understanding the weight of our sin helps us to recognize our desperate need for a Savior. Sin is deceptive, and our hearts are deceitful. Our hearts like to believe that our sin is "not that bad" or, at times, even "good." An example of this would be lying to a friend to avoid hurting their feelings. Not wanting to hurt someone is a good thing, but lying is still a sin, so this action is still sinful. The same is true when the actions seem "good," but the intention is sinful. One example is reading your Bible every day so that you can brag to all of your friends about it. Spending time in scripture is a good and right thing, but if the intention is pride and not growing in relationship with the Lord, this is still a sin. The truth is, however, that anything not done in faith is a sin (Romans 4:23).

If you are born again in Christ, the Holy Spirit lives in you (John 3:7). Because believers are filled with the Holy Spirit, we will always feel the weight of conviction for our sins at some point, even if that point is far removed from the sin itself or years later, as John 16:8 reminds us. Conviction is not to be confused with condemnation. The Holy Spirit does not condemn believers. Conviction is what some people may refer to as our conscience. Even non-believers have a conscience, but the Holy Spirit is a step further than this. The Holy Spirit is God living in us. The believer will feel conviction for things that the world praises (such as pride for doing the right thing or greed with what you earn). When you feel guilty for telling a lie or getting angry in traffic, this is the Holy Spirit convicting you of your sins. We also feel the Holy Spirit convicting us when we sin in bigger, more obvious ways. We should not confuse conviction in the Spirit with an unhealthy and condemning sense of guilt and shame.

How does this relate to our relationship with food? We should strive to be prayerful and discern what is conviction from the Holy Spirit in our lives and what is guilt and shame that comes from diet culture. The Spirit will not convict us of things that are not actually sinful. The Bible is clear about what constitutes obvious sin (see Galatians 5:19-21, James 4:17, Matthew 5:22-28, et al.). While there is less clarity around what is truly sinful regarding food, hopefully the Holy Spirit is beginning to open your eyes.

Romans 7:10 reminds us that sin promises life and happiness (the attractiveness of sin) but brings death and separation from God. Romans 7 continues to describe the human condition as we pursue Christlikeness and discusses the dilemma that even as we follow Jesus, we still tend to not understand our own sinful actions (Romans 7:15-20). We are tempted every day. The things we do not want to do, we do, and the good and right things that we desire, we do not do. We have the desire to do what is right, but not the ability to carry it out. As mentioned before, our actions themselves may not be sinful, or may even be good, but if the motivation is against God and rooted in ourselves, we are still in sin. As we understand the heaviness of our sin and how deeply it offends our perfect Father, we can be increasingly grateful for Jesus' sacrifice.

Because sin resides in our hearts and our heart posture dictates our actions, sin *does* relate to how we view food and our bodies. Therefore, wanting to go on a diet or engaging in disordered eating behaviors is usually the result of (sometimes hidden) sinful intentions. Disordered eating can also be the result of being sinned against and the overall effects of living in a broken world. For example, negative comments about your body made by loved ones, growing up in a food insecure household, or abuse against your body, all of which can lead to disordered eating. While it all is a result of a fallen world, and caused by original sin, the way someone has been sinned against can also perpetuate dieting and disordered eating behaviors. Studying sin, we see that any thought, behavior, or attitude that is rooted in more of ourselves than God is sinful. While pursuing health and stewarding your body in a way that honors God is a good and right thing, this can be a slippery slope to becoming idolatry. What occupies most of your thoughts and behaviors? Who is at the center of your motivations? Is it Christ and becoming more like Him, or is it changing your body to fit an ideal that is not found in scripture? Nowhere in the Bible does it say that we should feel guilty for eating certain foods after the New Covenant. Guilt has no place when it comes to eating a variety of foods, even foods that diet culture would say are "bad." We should only feel guilty for unrepentant sin. Eating to fuel your body and enjoying food is not sinful! At the heart of every desire is the question of whether your thoughts and behaviors support a Christ-enthroned life or a self-focused life.

The pursuit of perfection is common. Trying to be more Christlike is a good thing, but when it becomes all-consuming, or turns into perfectionism, it can become an idol. Matthew 5:48 says, *"You therefore must be perfect, as your heavenly Father is perfect."* This verse can be taken out of context to justify perfectionism, specifically as it relates to pursuing a "perfect bill of health." For example, counting grams of fat, carbohydrates, and protein to get the macronutrient balance "perfect." This is not what this verse means. During Jesus' time, there was no such thing as a nutrition facts label, so Jesus was not able to count everything to make it "perfect." Although recommendations can be helpful, there is no "one size fits all" for perfect eating. In one of Jesus' most famous teachings, the Sermon on the Mount (Matthew 5-7), He teaches how to live a righteous life. He preaches on a variety of topics (anger, lust, divorce, loving your enemies, and more), but His teaching can be summed up in verse 48. Verse 48 in The Message translation says: *"In a word, what I'm saying is, Grow up. You are kingdom subjects. Now, live like it. Live out your God-created identity. Live generously and graciously toward others, the way God lives toward you."* [A] We are to try to live a life that reflects Christ increasingly each day (sanctification), but we will never reach full perfection. Jesus alone was perfect. Though we can strive, we are not to try and replace God on the throne of our lives. This is a sin.

Pursuing health in a way that honors God is not sinful. However, even the word "health" is nuanced. Take some time here to consider your personal definition of health. If you were to write out a definition of health, what would you write? Often, when we think of health, we only think of physical health. But health encompasses so much more than that! Health can include physical, mental/emotional, spiritual, and relational well-being. Intuitive eating dietitian, Cara Harbstreet created an entire workbook on what "healthy eating" looks like for life.[2,B] One of the first activities in this workbook is to define health. Starting with physical health, you are asked to assess how you want to feel and what you consider to be an ideal quality of life. This is highly individualized, and two people will likely not have the exact same answers. Next, you are to assess your mental and emotional health and how you would define this. How do you honor your feelings and utilize the resources at your disposal? An example of this could be seeking counseling when you are in a season of stress. Another aspect of health Harbstreet asks you to define is your financial health. How would your financial situation be different if your health or eating habits changed? If you were not spending money on "diet foods" or other "health items," what would you do with that money instead? It goes on to define spiritual health. Knowing that health is multifaceted, we can begin to unpack what it truly means to be "healthy" and what this looks like for you. Finally, she asks you to assess your relational health. Being in a community is so important for growing your faith (1 John 1:7, Galatians 6:2, James 5:16, Proverbs 27:17, et. al). Dieting and disordered eating isolate us from community and interpersonal relationships. This is exactly what the enemy wants! As we isolate ourselves, we spend less time with God and others who know Him. Our time is spent focusing inward. In contrast, as you begin to put less focus on eating "perfectly," you can use that mental energy to connect more with Jesus. This is important because how we view food and our bodies impacts our faith.

Promoting physical health can look like eating in a way that feels good, listening to your body, and giving yourself permission to eat foods that satisfy hunger without guilt. This does not mean we should not eat "healthy foods" or throw out all we know about nutrition. While some foods are more nutrient-dense than others, guilt has no place when it comes to eating. Eating is *not* inherently sinful. Eating foods that have less nutritional value or are even labeled "bad" is *not* a sin, so you do *not* need to feel guilty for eating these foods. If you are thinking, "What about chronic illness? What if I need to follow a special diet for health reasons?" These scenarios are not included. If you need to avoid certain foods (for example, avoiding gluten if you have celiac disease or peanuts if you have a peanut allergy), you should respect your body by not eating those foods. Chapter 10 will go into more detail on listening to and respecting your body and how these are not mutually exclusive. In case you are thinking, "If I allow myself to eat whatever I want, whenever I want, I'll only ever eat ice cream and cookies," you are also not alone.

In the same way that you would grow tired and bored with broccoli and apples if you ate them every day, you would also grow tired and bored of your formerly forbidden foods if you allow yourself to have them without guilt. In the beginning, you may eat more of your off-limits foods, but over time, giving yourself unconditional permission to eat leads to more balance and variety. It is important to note here that this boredom with forbidden foods will only happen when you are fueling your body with adequate carbohydrates, proteins, and fats. It is normal to crave higher carbohydrate foods (quick energy) when you are not eating enough. Nutritional adequacy is so important, and you can eat all foods at all times without feeling guilty.

As mentioned above, mental and relational health are also important aspects of overall health. Contrary to popular belief, we are not in complete control of our mental health. Some individuals have lower blood levels of serotonin, which leads to clinical depression. Praise God for the common graces of medicine and counseling. Our mental health itself is not sinful either, but how we handle it can be. Our disappointment and depressive thoughts should not justify disobedience and permit sin. For example, "I am feeling really anxious. It's okay if I gossip," or "I'm feeling low; it's okay if I numb out with the overconsumption of alcohol." Anxiety, depression, or any other mental health issues, whether temporarily or chronically, are real struggles, but please do not forget to take this to the Lord in prayer and utilize the resources that you have available. Get connected to a local church and commit to being in a community with other believers. Eating disorders, depression and difficult intrusive thoughts thrive in isolation. Hebrews 10:24-25 reminds us of the importance of meeting with fellow believers. Relationships with other people who love Jesus are essential to pursuing overall health and well-being.

Prioritizing health as the most important value in your life and putting this over your relationship with the Lord (your *spiritual* health) is sinful. One way to see if health has become an idol is to reflect on these questions:

- Which do you feel more guilty about, skipping a day of going to the gym/not getting "enough steps," or skipping a quiet time?
- What percentage of your thoughts are about food or your body? What percentage of your thoughts are about God or spending time in prayer? If the first percentage is higher than the second, this might be an idol.
- Do you find yourself trying to eat "perfectly" based on the world's standards, yet you are not pursuing Christlikeness in the same way you are pursuing a perfect plate?
- Do you feel more guilt for eating "bad" food than you do for an actual sin (such as lust, anger, lying, etc.)?

Hebrews 4:16 says, *"let us then with confidence draw near to the throne of grace, that we may receive mercy and find grace to help in time of need."* If you find yourself in a sinful cycle of dieting and/or disordered eating, there is abounding grace for that. Jesus did not die for us to feel guilty for our sins that we repent of (or for us to feel guilty about eating in a way that is not sinful). He came to set us free (Romans 8:2). He covers all of our sins when we trust Him. Run to Jesus! Draw near to Him with confidence! Confess your sins and repent.[c]

. . .

PRAYER

Dear God,

Thank you for being so gracious and merciful to me. You tell us in Psalm 103:8 that you are slow to anger and abound in steadfast love. I confess that I sometimes put my pursuit of physical health over my nearness to You. Help me to put my physical health in its rightful place and help me to trust You in this. Draw near to me and show me your steadfast love.

In Jesus' name, amen.

FOOTNOTES:

A. The Message is a summary Bible translation that can be used alongside another translation, such as the English Standard Version, to help us understand the point and the main ideas of the passage. It should not be used as a stand-alone translation because it often leaves out important information in an effort to summarize scripture and help it make sense to modern readers.

B. Although this is a secular workbook, I (Anna Marie) would highly recommend it for anyone struggling to define health and wanting more practical tools for intuitive eating.

C. More on repentance will be discussed in chapter 6, as well as what this looks like practically.

SOURCES:

1. Grudem, W. A. *Systematic theology: An introduction to biblical doctrine*. Grand Rapids, Michigan. Zondervan Pub. House; 2000.

2. Harbstreet C. *Healthy Eating for Life: An Intuitive Eating Workbook to Stop Dieting Forever*. Althea Press; 2019.

5

THE GOSPEL

"For God so loved the world, that he gave his only Son, that whoever believes in Him should not perish but have eternal life. For God did not send His Son into the world to condemn the world, but in order that the world might be saved through Him."
~ John 3:16-17 (ESV)

AS WE BEGIN to scratch the surface of learning about ourselves, God's character, and our own sin, we need to make the connection of why all of these things matter, which is that Jesus came to set us free. He left His throne in Heaven with the Father to be with us in this broken world, and He consistently identifies with the outcasts and those society ignores.

Jesus understands what it is like to be in need. Leviticus 12:6-8 commanded that two offerings should be made after childbirth. One of the offerings was supposed to be a year-old blemish-free lamb. In verse 8, it makes the exception that if the woman cannot afford a lamb, two turtledoves will suffice. In Luke 2:22-24, Jesus was presented in the temple, and Mary and Joseph offered two turtledoves. Mary and Joseph could not afford much, yet this is where the Lord chose to come to us on earth. He lived a perfect life, died for our sins, was resurrected on the third day, and sits at the right hand of the Father. We can accept Christ as our Savior and be completely forgiven of our sins, but if we are not walking in freedom, it is difficult to accept the gospel for ourselves on a heart level. Walking in freedom means that we are living out the joy that is only found in Christ.[A] A question to ask ourselves is, do we actually believe that Jesus died for our sins and has the power to set us free from a life of bondage to disordered eating? When we are walking in slavery to food and body image struggles, we may not believe the entirety of the gospel applies to us.

The cost for all of our sins is death, but Jesus died so that we can live eternally with Him (Romans 6:23). Before sin entered the world, there was no death. When Adam and Eve sinned in the garden, they brought death into the world. God, being just, punishes everything evil that humans ever do with death. Thus, because of our sins, we deserve death, but Jesus died in our place to atone (or make amends) for our sins (1 John 2:2). No one can escape the human condition.

Before Jesus' death and resurrection, the Israelites (God's chosen people) had to make sacrifices to atone for their sins. Several types of sacrifices were required, such as a burnt offering, a wave offering, a peace offering, a purification offering, and a guilt offering. Depending on the sin or the time of year, the Israelites had to make sacrifices to be in right standing with God.[B] We no longer need to make these offerings because Jesus' sacrifice was enough once and for all! Eternal life is a free gift that is given to us when we accept Christ as our Savior. When we are offered this gift, we must receive it in full. In this particular case, it is important to think in an all-or-nothing manner. You either accept 100% of the free gift, or you do not accept it at all. You cannot accept 50% of the gift.

When the Israelites made an offering to atone for their sins, an animal had to die in their place. Now, instead of obtaining the best blemish-free lamb as a burnt offering, Jesus was Himself the perfect Lamb who offered Himself for us all (Revelation 5:9). Nothing we have done or will ever do can change what Jesus has already done for us on the cross. No sin that you have ever committed in the past or that you will commit in the future can separate you from the love of God (Romans 8:39).

During Jesus' earthly ministry, he preached that He came to fulfill the Law (Matthew 5:17). John 1:14 explains how Jesus dwelt among us and how He was the only Son of the Father. John 10:22-42 discusses how the religious leaders of the time did not want to believe that Jesus was the Christ and fulfillment of the Law, but Jesus was clear that He and the Father are One.

When Jesus died on the cross, He was in the tomb and dead for three days. On the third day, He rose from the dead (Luke 24:1-12), just as He said (Luke 9:22). Because of Jesus' sacrifice, although our physical bodies may perish, our souls will get to spend eternity with God (Romans 8:11, 2 Corinthians 4:16). We will have resurrected bodies and get to be with Jesus in paradise! Accepting the gospel not only means that you will have eternal life when you die, but it also means that you get to live your life right now in the abundance of joy that is found only in Jesus.

Receiving the gospel means living like we believe that Jesus' death and resurrection were enough to bring us from death in our sins to life in Christ. If we persist in our recurring patterns of sin voluntarily (willfully *choosing* sin over Jesus), it suggests that our hearts may not be fully embracing the gospel. When we *choose* to engage in disordered eating behaviors and align our hearts with the world's definition of and over prioritization of physical health, we may not believe that Jesus is enough for us.

The enemy likes to make us believe that we are "too far gone" or that our sins are "too much," and that we do not deserve the grace that is freely given to us. In one way, this is correct because we do not deserve grace (Romans 5:15-17). Grace is getting what we do not deserve. Imagine you are a college student, and your parents tell you they will pay for your school tuition as long as you pass all of your classes. But then you fail one class, and your parents still pay your tuition for the next semester. Your parents would be completely justified in not paying your tuition, but they decide to give you what is underserved. This is a *tiny* example of the grace that God gives to us. God would be justified in letting us die in our sins, but He shows us grace time and time again. But because of God's grace, we have unmerited favor. Mercy, on the other hand, is not getting what we actually deserve, or withholding punishment. If you are caught speeding but the police officer gives a warning rather than a deserved ticket, this is mercy. Because God loves us so much, He offers both His grace and mercy freely. When we believe the lie that our sin is too much, we are diminishing God's grace and mercy in our own lives.

This does not mean we ignore conviction: guilt can be good and right when it comes from the Holy Spirit and prompts us to run to the Father and ask for forgiveness. We should follow David's example in Psalm 139:23-24 and ask God to *"search [our] hearts and know [us]"* and make clear to us anyways we have sinned against Him. As soon as our sin is revealed, we should confess and repent.ᴬ Once we do this, our sin is forgiven! We should not walk in guilt and shame for sins that have already been forgiven. When God forgives us, we are set free from our guilt. While the enemy wants us to feel guilty forever (Revelation 12:10), God the Father sees Jesus when He looks upon those who have believed in Him. In the inevitable times when we find that we *still* feel guilty for sins that have already been confessed and forgiven, we can pray and meditate on Psalm 103:8-12, which reminds us that the Lord removes our sins from us and takes them away from us *"as far as the east is from the west."* We can also ask the Lord to restore the joy in us that is only found in Him (Psalm 51:12).

.   .   .

PRAYER

Dear God,

Thank You so much for the grace and mercy that you give us. We do not deserve this, yet You sent Your Son, Jesus to die so that we could spend eternity with You. You are a good and gracious Father. Help me to remember this when I feel guilty about things that are not sinful. Give me wisdom to discern the difference between my own sin and the ways that the enemy wants me to feel guilty when I am not in sin. Help me to believe that Jesus' death and resurrection are enough to cover my past, present, and future sins.

In Jesus' name, amen.

FOOTNOTES:

A. More on what it means practically to walk in the freedom of Christ is found in the next chapter. This chapter also covers the practice of confession and repentance.

B. For more on all of the sacrifices, see the entire book of Leviticus. While Leviticus can be a difficult read because of the specificity of all of the sacrifices, as well as the instructions for priests, it gives significance to Jesus fulfilling the Law.

6

FREEDOM IN CHRIST APPLIED

*"For freedom, Christ has set us free; stand firm, therefore, and
do not submit again to a yoke of slavery."*
~ Galatians 5:1 (ESV)

WE FREQUENTLY PERCEIVE freedom as our eternal freedom in
Heaven. Although true, this view of freedom is quite limited because
it neglects the reality that we have already been set free. The gospel is
less about getting us into Heaven and more about getting Heaven into
us *so that* we can walk in this freedom. In Romans 5:12-17, we see that
one offense (Adam's sin) subjected everyone to condemnation, but
the passage makes it very clear that grace has come for all people
through one man: Jesus Christ. Because of Jesus, we are no longer
subject to the Law.

Romans 6 beautifully portrays the tension of being made free by Jesus' blood but still sinning. The chapter begins with, "What shall we say then? Are we to continue in sin that grace may abound? By no means! How can we who died to sin still live in it?" (verses 1-2), then towards the end of the chapter we are called former "slaves of sin" (verse 20). Slavery is the bondage to a master. Slavery has been terribly corrupt throughout history, and likewise, slavery to sin corrupts our hearts. In Numbers 4, the Israelites were freed from slavery and bondage to Pharaoh. After being in bondage for years, it was not easy for them to adjust to their newfound freedom. Once released by Pharaoh, freedom did not mean ease for the Israelites, as they had to navigate what it looked like to establish a new life. Exodus 16:3 says that the Israelites complained to Moses and Aaron after being released, saying that they brought them out of Egypt to "die in the wilderness" and to "starve." At this point, the Israelites claimed that they would rather go back to slavery in Egypt than to trust God while in the desert with what He had planned for them. This was similarly seen in America's history when the Emancipation Proclamation was written. John Elmore commented on this saying "Jesus Christ our Lord has written an emancipation proclamation in Romans 6."[1] Sadly, God permitted them to wander in the desert for forty years due to their lack of submission and rose up the next generation who would be the ones actually able to enter the promised land. Similarly, if we demand to stay in slavery and bondage, God will allow it. If we submit and act on faith in God's promises, He will align our desires with His and will ultimately bring us His good purposes.

When we look at our lives, we can see a tension between freedom and bondage to sin. Maybe chapter 5 was the first time you heard of the gospel, and you feel like this freedom has been withheld from you. On the other hand, maybe you knew the freedom that was purchased for you on the cross, but not what it looks like to navigate this freedom in such a broken world. When Romans 6 introduces us as former slaves to sin, the apostle Paul asks the question of, *"What fruit were you getting at that time from the things of which you are now ashamed?"* (Romans 6:20). Think of the term fruit here as "benefit." When we sin, we believe that our way is better than God's way. Sin always over-promises and under-delivers.

So then, what *lasting* benefit is there from restricting food, obsessively exercising, or neglecting to take care of your body as beloved? A perceived benefit may be that restriction leads to weight loss, which makes you "more attractive" (more on this in chapter 16), which gains you more approval, etc., but what about the physical and behavioral consequences? Early physical signs of disordered eating may include feeling cold all the time, abdominal distress, fatigue, mental fog, sleep problems, and more. But these symptoms can progress into fainting, brittle hair and nails, infertility, osteoporosis, and electrolyte abnormalities, to name a few! What about some behavioral signs? There may be isolation from the preoccupied concern with eating in social settings, checking your body in the mirror or looking at pictures constantly to see if your body has changed, or purging, which can cause acid reflux, among other irreversible and long-term consequences. These are not listed to evoke fear, but they are listed to point out the stark reality of the consequences of eating disorders. Needless to say, there is not any eternal benefit to disordered eating. While it is important to be aware of these effects, having knowledge of these consequences does not necessarily lead to behavior and heart change.

Likewise, when we look back to the Garden of Eden in the book of Genesis, we see that merely knowledge of what to do and not do does not set us free. In other words, Adam and Eve knew God had instructed them to *"not eat of the fruit of the tree that is in the midst of the garden"* (Genesis 3:3), but they ate of it nonetheless. Knowing that we have been made in the image of God, how does that knowledge actually help us walk in freedom from the enslavement of negative body image? What does it practically look like to live in freedom but not abuse this grace already purchased for us?

The first step to being free is the recognition that something is not right. The fact that you have made it this far in this book shows that you have likely already recognized this. In the context of food and body image struggles, once you have taken that brave first step in acknowledging there is an unhealthy relationship with your body or food, a deeper dive can happen. Most of the time, disordered eating or eating disorders actually have nothing to do with the food itself. Eating disorders are not addictions to food or about the biological makeup of food.

Eating disorders are fueled by a negative cultural climate and underlying issues that push people harder and further into using dieting as a means of comfort or control.[2] Think of the classic iceberg analogy in Freudian theory; dieting, excessive exercise, and obsession with weight loss are on the top (ice that is seen), but perfectionism, past trauma, anxiety, genetics, emotional dysregulation, etc., lie underneath the surface (in the water where you cannot see). Any initial food or body image struggle may manifest itself in what is called a surface idol. Essentially, an idol is anything or anyone we give more love or worth to than God.

Simply put, *anything* can be an idol if we value it over God. A few surface idol examples could be an image idol, where you find value in how you look; a relationship idol, where you find value only if a certain person is attracted to you; and a suffering idol, which means you only feel worthy if you are in pain and thus feel justified to receive love. Other surface idols could include religion, work, materialism, or dependence (but we could go on!).

As mentioned earlier, with the iceberg, there is often something beneath the surface that is much bigger and more dangerous. Take, for instance, John. John loves running and makes it a priority to run most days. A few years ago, John tripped on a tree branch while running and busted his kneecap. John was unable to run for 9 weeks, per his doctor's recommendations. During those 9 weeks, he realized that when he wasn't running, he was engaging in other disordered behaviors to avoid weight gain. His thoughts were often about manipulating his body so that he would appear the same pre-injury as he did post-injury. After about 4 weeks, John decided he "felt fine" and went for a jog. John re-injured his kneecap and had to rest for several additional weeks, but his heart was set on running. Even though it appeared to be about enjoyment, when running was taken away from him, he was able to uncover the idol of control (in this case, controlling his body) underneath the love of running. This is a deeper source of idolatry.

The four source idols hide themselves much more subversively yet oftentimes drive all our other idols. These include comfort, power, control, or approval/significance.[3] Idols often have deep roots, especially roots from how we were raised.[A] If we are not purposeful in cultivating the deep roots of our hearts and only touch the surface, we will replace one bad habit (or sin) with another. For example, someone with a comfort idol may replace using food for comfort with alcohol for comfort to numb their feelings. Where we root our heart determines our fruit (think back to Romans 6:21), so we must rightly root our hearts.

A helpful tool that guides you in searching your heart is using a Fruit to Root tree derived from Jeff Vanderstelt in his book Gospel Fluency.[4] This exercise is similar to the iceberg analogy in that it helps you discover what is beneath the surface of your thoughts and behaviors. At the top, you start with a rotten fruit (behavior, thought, or action that is disobedient to God). From here, you "go down" the tree to ask yourself, "Who am I?" When you ask yourself this, you are asking who you believe yourself to be (the lie you are believing about yourself). Then, at the bottom, ask yourself, "What lies am I believing about God?"

This part reveals the current condition of your heart. But remember, God already knows every thought you have (Psalm 139:1-6), so you can confess these lies you are believing to Him. That is a huge step towards freedom. Romans 8:1-2 reminds us, *"There is therefore now no condemnation for those who are in Christ Jesus. For the law of the Spirit of life has set you free in Christ Jesus from the law of sin and death."* It is a beautiful thing to become more concerned with your inward spiritual condition (your heart towards God) rather than your outward appearance. There is a caveat here, though. If all you do is confess but not repent, you are more likely to allow other sinful habits to grow where the weed was.

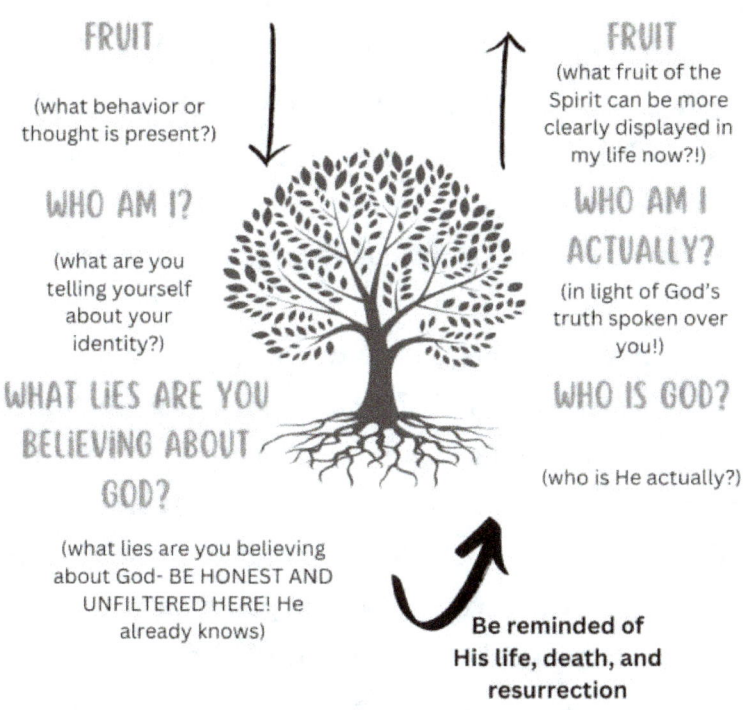

FRUIT

(what behavior or thought is present?)

WHO AM I?

(what are you telling yourself about your identity?)

WHAT LIES ARE YOU BELIEVING ABOUT GOD?

(what lies are you believing about God- BE HONEST AND UNFILTERED HERE! He already knows)

FRUIT

(what fruit of the Spirit can be more clearly displayed in my life now?!)

WHO AM I ACTUALLY?

(in light of God's truth spoken over you!)

WHO IS GOD?

(who is He actually?)

Be reminded of His life, death, and resurrection

For a more thorough understanding of gospel fluency with a fruit to root tree, we highly recommend Jeff Vanderstelt's book. For our purposes however, we have created an example as it relates to food and body image. Let us say the "fruit" or "behavior" is that I am editing every picture I post on Instagram to manage my appearance out of shame with the way I look. Under the "who am I?" pervasive lies that I am telling myself is that I am "bigger than my friends," "never going to attract a guy," and "unable to hold a steady weight." I am believing the lie that by editing a picture, maybe a guy will be more likely to slide into my DMs like the rest of my friends. I think that my family members will make another comment about my changing weight. I am also embarrassed to stand out from the way the rest of my friends look. Next, I write out the lies I believe about God. In this specific case, I write, "I believe that God is withholding good from me, is untrustworthy in the way He made my biological cues, and that He will never deliver me from the comparison and fear I have around peers and family." Then, when I look at Jesus' life, I am reminded that He constantly sought out the outcasts. He did not look toward the outward appearances of man. Jesus was single and fully content and complete in Himself. Jesus wholeheartedly pursued the things of the Father. In His death, Jesus foresaw my struggles with envy of others' bodies, bitterness toward family, lack of belief in God, self-sufficiency and pride and chose to be the atonement for my sins. When He rose again three days later, He demonstrated power over Satan, sin, and death. So, when I am reminded of the gospel, I can now answer "Who is God?" rightly. I am reminded that God is indeed powerful enough to deliver me from comparison and fear. God is gracious in giving me the good gift of the community around me. He knows exactly what I need when I need it, He withholds no good, and He made no mistake in creating me. Considering the truth about God, I realize that I am actually sought after by the King of the universe, and thus, I now realize I do not need to edit every picture I post. I can have peace knowing that pictures are momentary shots that will ultimately collect dust. I can focus my attention on the joy of the moment of the pictures rather than the pictures themselves.

Repentance is the act of turning away from your sin *and* turning toward Christ. Because we continue to sin and fall short of the glory of God everyday (Romans 3:23), we need continual repentance to walk in lasting freedom. We also know repentance is not just a suggestion for us, but it is an actual command written throughout scripture. In Acts 2:38, Peter, one of Jesus' disciples, commands, *"Repent and be baptized every one of you in the name of Jesus Christ for the forgiveness of your sins, and you will receive the gift of the Holy Spirit."* There is not anything we can do to save ourselves. The passage then tells us that on that day, 3,000 souls were saved. The Lord does indeed produce great fruit in the lives around us when we come to him humbly with a repentant heart, but fruit is never the goal. Though the gospel should be shared with others, the gospel is also about our inward transformation.

We see in 2 Corinthians 7:10 that, *"Godly grief produces a repentance that leads to salvation without regret, whereas worldly grief produces death."* It should hurt our hearts to know that our sin hurts the heart of God, but remember, we should not feel shame for this. Instead, our affection for the sacrifice of Jesus should all the more be stirred! Hallelujah! Likewise, we do not need to feel guilt for what has been confessed and forgiven. Shame is the idea of feeling "unclean or dirty." Guilt, on the other hand, is the feeling when we violate a *moral* standard or law. Thus, it is important to distinguish between true guilt and false guilt. Say, for example, you feel guilty after lying to your parents or spouse, running a red light, or stealing something from a friend. That sense of guilt may be helpful in stirring you into the action of confessing because it is a conscious decision not to do those things. False guilt, conversely, occurs when we create our own moral code. Think about some food or exercise rules you have made for yourself (it may even be helpful to write these down). A few examples may include (but are not limited to):

- I must exercise if I eat dessert
- I need to burn X calories to be able to eat all of my meals and snacks
- I can't eat after a specific time at night
- I am not allowed to eat breakfast if I had a big dinner the night before
- I must have fruit or vegetables at every meal
- I can't drink anything with calories
- I can only have one serving of packaged foods every day
- I must take the stairs only
- I must have a plan with food every day and cannot deviate from my plan

These rules may feel safe and compelling, but they ultimately cannot produce fruit in your life. The actions we take after repentance are not *to receive* God's grace, but because we *already have* received God's grace. Sometimes, the idea of true guilt can be known as conviction.

As you have begun to acknowledge unhealthy behavioral patterns that exist in your life with food, exercise, and your body, you also may have already begun to brainstorm some surface and source idols you see in your day-to-day thoughts and behaviors. If you have not yet done so, consider taking some time to do that now. Through confession of the lies you are believing about yourself and about God and the brainstorming of rules you have created for yourself, it is evident that *"the desires of the flesh are against the Spirit, and the desires of the Spirit are against the flesh"* (Galatians 5:17).

The weight loss industry desires your money, not your freedom. This is evident through the endless weight loss plans and centers, diet books, and supplements that keep us contributing to this multibillion-dollar industry. The more insecure we are, the more diet companies profit. Beauty standards change from generation to generation and year to year. As they continue to evolve, we are perpetually being marketed new things. If this has not been repeated enough, we must not conform to the world. Society may portray the next diet as freedom from feeling "tired all the time" and "gross in your body," but in reality, this is lowering standards for yourself because you are allowing those who do not even know you to tell you about your worth and what you need to fix. What comes before Galatians 5:17, though, is quite remarkable. The Scripture states, *"Walk by the Spirit, and you will not gratify the desires of the flesh"* (Galatians 5:16). Think about the word "walk". How do you physically walk? You put one step in front of the other repeatedly - boom! You are walking. In this same manner is the Christian life: the temptations will not stop. Social media and technology are here to stay. Marketers still want your money. Research is forever evolving. So we must also walk through the trenches, upstream of diet culture, hand in hand with Jesus.

. . .

PRAYER

Father God,

Thank You for sending your Son Jesus to set me free. Please help me to walk in the truth that I am no longer enslaved to my sin. Convict me of my fleshly desires in my heart that lie beneath my disordered patterns. Reveal to me the idols I am placing over You, Lord. I ask that you guide me in uprooting the lies I believe. Increase my faith and trust in You. I shall put on the full armor of God so that I can withstand evil. I shall not gratify the desires of the flesh. Jesus, I desire to walk in your ways of righteousness with all parts of my life, and this includes my behaviors toward food and body. Grant me freedom from my struggles today.

In Jesus' name, amen.

FOOTNOTES:

A. For more on the family of origin and how our idols are rooted in our upbringing, please see chapter 7.

SOURCES:

1. Elmore, J. *Freedom Starts Today: Overcoming Struggles and Addictions One Day at a Time*. Grand Rapids, Michigan: Baker Books; January 19, 2021.
2. Costin C, Grabb GS. *8 Keys to Recovery from an Eating Disorder: Effective Strategies from Therapeutic Practice and Personal Experience (8 Keys to Mental Health)*. W. W. Norton & Company; November 7, 2011.
3. Keller T. *Counterfeit Gods: The Empty Promises of Money, Sex, and Power, and the Only Hope That Matters*. Riverhead Books; October 20, 2009.
4. Vanderstelt J. *Gospel Fluency: Speaking the Truths of Jesus into the Everyday Stuff of Life*. Crossway; February 28, 2017.

7

INTERNAL INFLUENCES

Impact of Trauma

*"The Lord is near to the brokenhearted and
saves the crushed in spirit."*
~Psalm 34:18 (ESV)

UP TO THIS point, we have laid out the significance of being made in the image of God, examined who God truly is and what sin is, looked at how sin corrupts us, recognized our need for the gospel, *and* we have understood how Jesus sets us free. Now, we will take some time to investigate a few barriers that may exist in this struggle, whether that be mental, emotional, or physical barriers.

Trauma is "when suffering overwhelms normal human coping."[1]

Trauma may impact someone's struggle with disordered eating. Similarly, eating disorders themselves can cause trauma to our physical bodies. While the practical details of the different types of traumas are beyond the scope of this book, it is important to discuss the need for taking a trauma-informed approach to eating disorder recovery. This is because eating disorders are usually not about the food itself but what underlies the behavior (though there are medical consequences to eating disorders).[2] Looking at just one example, trauma can result in someone's loss of physical connection to their own body, leading to difficulty with interoceptive awareness. Interoceptive awareness is an awareness of what is going on internally, like hunger-fullness cues, thirst, and physical pain.[3] This is a God-given gift to us for survival; however, when someone experiences a sense of disturbed safety from traumatic circumstances, awareness may shift away from their internal state and toward the external state out of a perceived need for self-protection. The body is hypervigilant.

Other possible results of trauma include dissociation from one's emotions or an overall loss of trust. People may begin to believe that they cannot trust their intuition, which may make their ability to trust in their bodies feel unmanageable, thus triggering an eating disorder as a form of control or self-soothing. Yet another (though far from the last) response to trauma is a sense of shame by the victim. Shame, as a result of emotional or verbal abuse, may lead to an urge to control whatever one can, internalizing the words and opinions of others, and believing false things about one's body.

It is all very complex, but the wirings of our body's response to trauma point us to the incredible design of our body that God created in us. Reactions can be both immediate and delayed. Our body may physically respond with nausea and gastrointestinal distress, fatigue, or elevated blood pressure to kick us into survival mode, telling us that something is off (sympathetic nervous system). Our mind may respond to this with disturbed sleep and appetite. Emotional reactions like guilt, anxiety, and feeling out of control may be exacerbated. Lastly, cognitive reactions that become more common are negative rumination (dwelling on negative thoughts) and distortion of things, like our bodies.

Even though He does not have the same human limitations as us because of His dual nature as both man and God, Jesus, our Savior, is not a stranger to trauma. Jesus was betrayed by a friend, mocked, and crucified (Mark 15). We see other examples throughout scripture of those who experienced trauma and the hope that the gospel brings in the midst of their trouble.[4] Mary and Martha witnessed the death of their ill brother, Lazarus (John 11). David had Saul break into his home and try to kill him (1 Samuel 18:6-16). David had an affair with Bathsheba and an unexpected pregnancy, and then Bathsheba had to deal with the loss of her husband at the hands of David (2 Samuel 11). Lot allowed his daughters to be taken advantage of sexually (Genesis 19:8). The Egyptians *"made the people of Israel work as slaves and made their lives bitter with hard service, in mortar and brick, and in all kinds of work in the field. In all their work, they ruthlessly made them work as slaves"* (Exodus 1:13-14). Trauma as a result of brokenness is not new to this world. It has been present since the fall. The Lord is the hope through it all, for He claims to be *"near to the brokenhearted and [saves] the crushed in spirit"* (Psalm 34:18).

If trauma is a part of your story, what are some ways you can respond? The first step is lamenting the injustice you experienced. Let this be repaid by the *"wrath of God, for it is written, 'Vengeance is mine, I will repay'"* (Romans 12:19). The book *Dark Clouds, Deep Mercy: Discovering the Grace of Lament* by Mark Vroegop lays out the following steps to lament through observing the scriptures. You begin by turning to God. Next, bring God your honest complaint, ask boldly for God to act, and finish by recalling God's character and previous faithfulness, so choosing to trust.[5] Psalm 55 is a great example of how to lament. In fact, one-third of the Psalms are lamenting Psalms!

For a second practical application, please take note of your triggers and build awareness of them. Examples of triggers from physical eating disorder trauma may be hearing the doctor call out your weight, receiving specific body comments on social media, or watching someone else count calories or macros. After you have identified your triggers, make a plan for how to try to cope with triggers for the inevitable times they arise. Most importantly, invite the Lord into this! God *"will not let you be tempted beyond your ability, but with the temptation, he will also provide the way of escape, that you may be able to endure it"* (1 Corinthians 10:13). Speak with a counselor to learn effective coping and grounding exercises. This may help with interoceptive awareness, too.

Lastly, be patient, for it is a fruit of the Spirit (Galatians 5:22)! Healing takes time. Whether you yourself have experienced trauma or a close friend or family member, follow through in obedience to 1 Thessalonians 5:14, which says, *"admonish the idle, encourage the fainthearted, help the weak, be patient with them all."* Whether or not you have experienced trauma from within your family, your family of origin still has a huge impact on you (for better or for worse). It is important not to find our identity in situations that have happened to us. Instead, we should seek insight into how our past has impacted our present curiously and compassionately.

Impact of Family of Origin

"For you did not receive the spirit of slavery to fall back into fear, but you have received the Spirit of adoption as sons, by whom we cry, 'Abba! Father!' The Spirit himself bears witness with our spirit that we are children of God."
~ Romans 8:15 (ESV)

FAMILY OF ORIGIN typically refers TO those that had a significant role in someone's development. We will briefly examine the potential impacts of a mother and father; however, we also recognize that not everyone grew up with a biological mother or father. Hence, this could refer to the people who raised you as a child.

Attachment theory is the concept that individuals develop attachment styles based on relationships with their early caregivers. Four styles currently exist: secure attachment, attachment anxiety, attachment avoidance, and disorganized attachment.[6] Research has shown that disordered behaviors are correlated with emotional dysregulation. Disordered eating is a disordered behavior and a precursor to eating disorders. Connecting the two, previous research has indicated that emotional dysregulation contributes to the onset and maintenance of an eating disorder.[7] The way in which children and adolescents learn emotional regulation skills is largely influenced by parental attachment relationships.[8] Specifically, mothers are the parental figure more frequently sought out for safe haven, or a sense of security,[9] as this is usually an infant's first connection.[9,A] In a study examining mother-daughter attachment in adolescents' effect on disordered eating prevalence into young adulthood, more secure attachment with a mother was found to significantly decrease the daughter's likelihood of engaging in binge eating ($p<0.01$), compensatory behaviors ($p<0.05$), and fasting/skipping meals ($p<0.001$).[9,B] A longitudinal study looking at depressive symptoms as a mediator between mother-daughter insecure attachment and disordered eating behaviors discovered that insecure mother-daughter attachment significantly predicted more depressive symptoms in the daughter ($p<0.001$, $p<0.001$, $p<0.05$). This, in turn, significantly predicted more disordered eating ($p<0.01$, $p<0.05$, $p<0.001$) at each two-year time interval through adolescence (10 to 12, 12 to 14, and 14 to 16 years of age).[10]

A third study investigated emotional reactivity, difficulty regulating emotions, parental attachment, and disordered eating and reported that insecure mother-daughter attachment significantly predicted emotional regulation difficulties among the daughter ($p<0.01$). This third study also found significant mediation from mother-daughter attachment to disordered eating through the daughter's regulation of emotions ($p=0.003$).[11] Similar results have been found consistently throughout other studies, including mediators like negative spirals or thought patterns and stress. Though it cannot be stated that mother-daughter insecure attachment *causes* disordered eating or eating disorders, there *is* a positive association.

In discussing these results, we should be cautious not to shift blame onto external circumstances for behaviors and struggles; rather, this research should be viewed as a gift to us. Our flesh, rooted in sinful self-righteousness, longs for error to be on anyone else but us. To be clear, parents *do not* directly cause eating disorders, but they can contribute to the development of disordered eating. With that said, investigating developmental and psychological research allows us to extend grace to ourselves and others and further recognize the imperfect world in which we live. Brokenness in relationships was not a part of God's design when He formed the world. Hallelujah, there will be no more brokenness in the New Jerusalem (Revelation 21:4).

When it comes to our relationships with earthly fathers, it is similarly tempting to blame them for the wrong views we have and lies we believe about our Heavenly Father.[A] However, this should not be so either. David Powlison, a gospel teacher, counselor, and executive director of the Christian Counseling and Educational Foundation, wrote, "the human agent (like our father), is certainly significant, but it always remains secondary."[12] God should always be the primary focus of our lives! Once again, as much as we may want to, we cannot draw causal statements and attribute blame. James warns us of the temptation of victim mentality in questioning us with, *"What causes quarrels and what causes fights among you? Is it, not this, that your passions are at war within you?"* (James 4:1). There is a spiritual realm that we do not see. Certainly, there are people with "bad parents" who have a great relationship with God, AND there are people with "good parents" who have a rotten view of God.[12] But ultimately, we know how God feels about us and His true character because He tells us in His Word. The Word of God must dictate the way we perceive God and not our personal experiences. If you are currently struggling with this, take hope in 2 Corinthians 4:6 as a prayer for your heart because God *"has shone in our hearts to give the light of the knowledge of the glory of God in the face of Jesus Christ."*

Ultimately, the blood of Christ unites the Family of God together. Believers residing in the United States, China, and Africa have more in common with one another than with a biological family who do not believe in Christ (Acts 2:44). Though the Family of God is far from perfect, we do get spiritual mothers and fathers. In Paul's ministry to the Thessalonians, he compared ministry to nurturing care like a nursing mother and encouragement and exhortation from a father (1 Thessalonians 2:7-12). If a mother and/or father were not compassionate in their care toward you, the Lord has promised, *"I will not forget you. Behold, I have engraved you on the palms of my hands; your walls are continually before me"* (Isaiah 49:15-16).

. . .

PRAYER

Dear God,

Forgive me for not seeing the entirety of Your character. You are a good Father to me. Continue to help my unbelieving heart believe in this promise. You will never fail me. When I feel the tension between myself and my family, remind me you put me in my family for a specific plan and purpose. Would you reconcile any wounds between my family members and I, too?

In Jesus' name, amen.

FOOTNOTES:

A. We acknowledge that not everyone knows or is known by their biological mother or biological father. This is an analysis of the research and current data, and if this information is difficult for you to read, please discuss this with your counselor.

B. The p-value is the likelihood that differences observed between one variable, and another are due to chance or are random. A statistically significant p-value is anything <0.05

SOURCES:

1.   Langberg D. *Suffering and the Heart of God: How Trauma Destroys and Christ Restores.* New Growth Press; September 15, 2015.

2.   Seubert AJ, Virdi P. *Trauma-Informed Approaches to Eating Disorders.* Springer Publishing Company, LLC; August 17, 2018.

3. Weir K. What is interoception, and how does it affect mental health? 5 questions for April Smith. *Monitor on Psychology.* April 1, 2023. https://www.apa.org/monitor/2023/04/sensations-eating-disorders-suicidal-behavior. Accessed May 20, 2024.

4. Beltran B. Understanding Trauma. Powerpoint presented at: The Austin Stone Recovery Workshop; March 25, 2023; Austin, TX.

5.   Vroegop M. *Dark Clouds, Deep Mercy: Discovering the Grace of Lament.* Crossway; March 21, 2019.

6.   Bowlby J. Attachment and loss: Retrospect and prospect. American *Journal of Orthopsychiatry*. 1982;52(4):664-678. doi:https://doi.org/10.1111/j.1939-0025.1982.tb01456.x

7.   Cortés-García L, Takkouche B, Seoane G, Senra C. Mediators linking insecure attachment to eating symptoms: A systematic review and meta-analysis. *PLoS One*. 2019;14(3):e0213099. Published 2019 Mar 7. doi:10.1371/journal.pone.0213099

8.   Negrini LS. Handbook of Attachment, Third Edition: Theory, research, and clinical applications. Jude Cassidy and Phillip R. Shaver (Eds.), New York: Guilford Press, 2016, 1,068 pp., ISBN 978-1-4625-2529-4. *Infant Mental Health Journal*. 2018;39(5):618-620. doi:https://doi.org/10.1002/imhj.21730

9.   Hazzard VM, Miller AL, Bauer KW, Mukherjee B, Sonneville KR. Mother–child and father-child connectedness in adolescence and disordered eating symptoms in young adulthood. *Journal of Adolescent Health*. 2020;66(3):366-371. doi:https://doi.org/10.1016/j.jadohealth.2019.09.019

10.   Cortés-García L, Viddal KR, Wichstrøm L, Senra C. Mediating role of depressive symptoms linking insecure attachment and disordered eating in adolescents: A multi-wave longitudinal study. *Development and Psychopathology*. Published online September 15, 2020:1-13. doi:https://doi.org/10.1017/s0954579420001029

11.   Vaydich JL, Carpenter TP, Schwark JK, Molina L. Disordered eating among college students: The effects of parental attachment and the mediating role of emotion dysregulation. *Journal of*

American College Health. Published online December 1, 2020:1-8. doi:https://doi.org/10.1080/07448481.2020.1846045

12. Powlison, D. What if Your Father Didn't Love You? - CCEF. https://www.ccef.org/jbc-article/what-if-your-father-didnt-love-you . Published 2016. Accessed June 3, 2024.

8

EXTERNAL INFLUENCES

Social Determinants of Health and Scarcity Eating

"I pray that all may go well with you and that you may be in good health, as it goes well with your soul."
~3 John 1:2 (ESV)

IT WOULD DO all of us a disservice to discuss nutrition and disordered eating without addressing food insecurity. Food insecurity is defined as a limited or uncertain ability to acquire or consume an adequate quality or sufficient quantity of food in socially acceptable ways.[1] In 2017, 40 million US individuals were food insecure. That is 1 in 8 people![2] In children, however, this is seen in 1 out of 6. Health and developmental conditions associated with childhood food insecurity include aggression and anxiety, poor glycemic control, "obesity," mental health problems, and iron deficiency anemia, to name a few. Those with great poverty typically struggle with both food insecurity and hunger. The 2020 U.S. Department of Health and Human Services (HHS) Poverty Guidelines for household income was $12,760 for a household of one and $26,200 for a household of four, to provide an example. Additionally, those with the highest rates of "obesity" are among those with the greatest poverty. This is multifactorial.

The metabolic and psychosocial stress in adults that comes with food insecurity leads to behavioral and emotional problems, reduced work capacity, poor academic achievement and focus, functional impairments, and health complications. Because of this, our body's natural survival tendency is to stretch food dollars by maximizing caloric intake to ward off hunger and overeating when food *is* available. This starvation to overeating cycle, or the feast and famine cycle, is seen in weight cycling with yo-yo diets in individuals who *have* access to food. This yo-yo weight cycling is part of the "obesity" paradox.

Our bodies are biologically set to fight against starvation (thank you, Lord!). When in chronic hunger, the basal metabolic rate (BMR) decreases. BMR is the energy it takes to maintain basic life functions like pumping blood, breathing, and sleeping. As hunger persists, the body's hormones are thrown into compensatory mechanisms. Our bodies have three major hormones released to signal satiety, but we only have one hormone that needs to be released to initiate hunger: ghrelin. The second our brain senses our stomach is empty; ghrelin will be secreted. This opposes the effects of dieting. Additionally, leptin, a satiety-signaling hormone, drops exponentially in periods of fasting (or starvation). These levels decrease much quicker than the body fat stores are depleted, once again as a protective measure to our body's set-point.

Those who deal with food insecurity often lack access to nutrient-dense foods. Foods that society demonizes and labels as "bad" are the food these people have access to and can afford. Additionally, those with limited access to foods often have an inadequate intake of energy, protein, vitamins, and minerals. The combination of these two can result in malnutrition and "obesity." Therefore, when reading literature about "obesity," it is crucial to pay attention to confounding variables like food insecurity. Because there are these confounding variables, we cannot draw causal statements from certain foods being the "reason for the obesity epidemic." Humans should never be ashamed of eating what is available and accessible.

Another common misconception is that malnutrition means a "small weight." This is far from the truth. In reality, someone could be classified in the BMI range of "overweight or obese" and still be considered malnourished due to other factors that are not usually considered, like vitamin and mineral status (deficiencies).[3] Malnutrition can be starvation-related, acute disease/injury-related, and chronic disease-related. While overall weight loss can be included in one of the criteria to diagnose malnutrition, other factors observed include grip strength, fluid accumulation, muscle mass loss, overall energy intake, and subcutaneous fat loss.[4]

It is also important to understand what true health is. As previously mentioned in chapter 4, health is not merely the absence of disease or infirmity; rather, it is measured more holistically through someone's internal health. To go a bit more in-depth, one working definition of health is that health "is a state of complete physical, mental and social well-being."[5] A second definition from a community nutrition researcher said, "A healthy individual has the physical, mental, and spiritual capacity to live, work, and interact joyfully with other human beings."[1]

When we zoom out and think about what has shaped our own view of health, a helpful model to use is the social-ecological model (SEM) of health behavior created by psychologist Urie Bronfenbrenner.[6] This looks at the nature of people's interactions with their surrounding physical and sociocultural environments. This starts with the individual (knowledge, attitudes, and beliefs) and gradually broadens to interpersonal relationships (family, friends, and associations), institutional/organizational impacts (policies), the community (social norms), and then finally, structures/policies and systems (local, state, and federal).

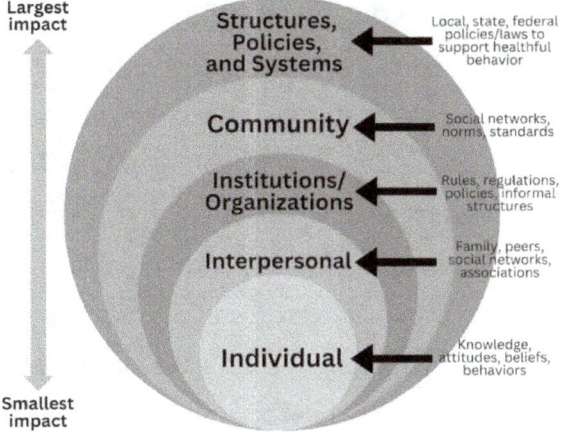

SOCIAL ECOLOGICAL MODEL
(SEM) OF HEALTH BEHAVIOR

Largest impact

Structures, Policies, and Systems — Local, state, federal policies/laws to support healthful behavior

Community — Social networks, norms, standards

Institutions/ Organizations — Rules, regulations, policies, informal structures

Interpersonal — Family, peers, social networks, associations

Individual — Knowledge, attitudes, beliefs, behaviors

Smallest impact

Adapted from Center for Disease Control and Prevention (CDC), The Social Ecological Model

Another model we must understand is social determinants of health (SDOH). When it comes to health, we know there are some fixed factors like age, sex, race, and genetics, but there are also *some* modifiable factors. SDOH are conditions in the environments where people are born, live, learn, work, play, and worship that affect a wide range of health, functioning, and quality of life outcomes and risks.[7] This is composed of five different categories. First, a category of SDOH is education access and quality. It has been proven that what someone learns up to age six profoundly impacts them later in life. This includes early childhood education, enrollment in higher education, language and literacy, public health outreach, and vocational training. We also know that education access can work hand in hand with employment later in life, a factor in economic stability. The second category of SDOH includes healthcare access and quality.

In America, 9% are uninsured, which is about 1 in 10 people![8] The concept of quality and access to healthcare includes health disparities, health literacy, cultural competency of healthcare providers, stress management, medical self-care, and safety practices. We know that many employment opportunities may provide some insurance; therefore, if education levels impact someone's ability to get a job, access to healthcare may also be a struggle. A third category of SDOH is the neighborhood and built environment, which, unfortunately, can often be impacted by where you can afford to live. This includes public safety and transportation, walkability (streetlights, sidewalks), parks and recreation spaces nearby and available, the climate, zip code, environmental conditions (pollution, etc.), safe water, and access to fresh food options. Some places are considered to be food deserts, which means there is a limited number of food retailers that provide fresh produce and groceries at affordable prices.[9] Other places are considered to be food swamps, which are areas with a high density of fast and convenience foods relative to more nutrient-dense food options.[10]

While fast and convenience foods have a place in a balanced diet, it is still important to have a variety available, and people in some environments may not have this freedom. The fourth SDOH category takes into account the social and community context of health. This includes cultural beliefs and attitudes, social and faith-based networks, legal services, food assistance programs available, government structure and policy, communication engagement, discrimination, and media messages. The fifth and final category of SDOH is economic stability, which ties into all the other components (employment status, income levels, presence of debt, and assets/expenses).

Given the above, it is important to have a more holistic lens when thinking about how we interpret research and health. Before healthcare providers ever make recommendations to people, it is imperative that they first look at what people can access. It is time for the healthcare industry to realize that a thinner body does not prevent chronic diseases, and a larger body does not cause them. There are many factors at play in individual lives.

. . .

PRAYER

Dear God,

In your perfect provision for me, would I be reminded that I brought nothing into this world, and I cannot take anything out of this world. Help me to be content if I have food on the table and clothes on my body. And help me be more aware of the ways in which I can serve those around me who may have limited access to food.

In Jesus' name, amen.

SOURCES:

1. Boyle, M. A. *Community Nutrition in Action*. 8th Edition. Cengage Learning; 2022.

2. Landry M. Associations between diet quality, vegetable availability and access, and food security in low-income children. Dissertation. University of Texas at Austin; 2019.

3. World Health Organization. Malnutrition. https://www.who.int/news-room/fact-sheets/detail/malnutrition. Published March 1, 2024.

4. Skipper A. Malnutrition coding. In Skipper A (ed). *Nutrition Care Manual*. Chicago, IL: Academy of Nutrition and Dietetics; 2012.

5. Constitution of the World Health Organization. www.who.int. https://www.who.int/about/governance/constitution#:~:text=WHO%20remains%20firmly%20committed%20to

6. Ewald DR, Orsini MM, Strack RW. The path to good health: Shifting the dialogue and promoting social ecological thinking. *SSM - Population Health*. 2023;22:101378. doi:https://doi.org/10.1016/j.ssmph.2023.101378

7. Healthy People 2030, U.S. Department of Health and Human Services, Office of Disease Prevention and Health Promotion. Retrieved from https://odphp.health.gov/healthypeople/objectives-and-data/social-determinants-health

8. Berchick, E.R. Hood, E., and Barnett, J. Health insurance coverage in the United States 2017. https://www.census.gov/content/dam/Census/library/publi

cations/2018/demo/p60-264.pdf. Published September 2017.

9. Dutko P, Ploeg M, Farrigan T. Characteristics and influential factors of food deserts. *United States Department of Agriculture;* 2012. https://www.ers.usda.gov/webdocs/publications/45014/30 940_err140.pdf

10. Cooksey-Stowers K, Schwartz MB, Brownell KD. Food swamps predict obesity rates Better than food deserts in the United States. *Int J Environ Res Public Health.* 2017;14(11):1366. Published 2017 Nov 14. doi:10.3390/ijerph14111366

9

FOOD

Jesus is the Bread of Life

"Jesus said to them, 'I am the bread of life; whoever comes to me shall not hunger, and whoever believes in me shall never thirst.'"
~ John 6:35 (ESV)

JOHN 6:22-59 TEACHES us that Jesus is our Bread of Life, and He is truly all we need. As He taught these things, some people were confused, yet others understood. While food fuels our bodies, Jesus nourishes our souls. After Jesus finished His miracle of feeding the five thousand with only five loaves of bread and two fish (John 6:1-15), He walked on water to catch up with His disciples in their boat (John 6:16-21). As Jesus and His disciples crossed the sea, the crowd got in their own boats and followed, desiring more of Jesus and the blessings He could provide. Jesus could see the motivation of their hearts, and so He rebuked them, acknowledging that they followed Him not because they saw signs, but because they "ate their fill of the loaves" (John 6:26). The people were following Jesus not because they wanted more of Him, but because they wanted more of what He could do for them. How often do we find ourselves doing the same? We pray to God, promising that if He just gives us what we want, we will go to church every Sunday, or we will do whatever we think it is that He wants. We can so easily want more of Jesus because of His blessings. While this specific story seems like something that we would never do, we often follow the same pattern.

Jesus goes on in John 6:27 to say, *"Do not work for the food that perishes, but for the food that endures to eternal life, which the Son of Man will give to you."* While food is important for the nourishment of our physical bodies, Jesus is our eternal fuel. He gives us Himself and fills us up in ways that food cannot. Jesus is what we need. The people then ask Jesus what they must do to get this eternal food (John 6:28), and He responds that they must believe in His Son whom He sent (John 6:29). God reveals Himself to us so that we may believe that Jesus is our salvation and that He is all that we need. Jesus then reminds His followers of how God provided manna for their ancestors to eat in the wilderness (John 6:31-33).

For forty years, the Israelites wandered in the wilderness after escaping slavery in Egypt, yet the Lord rained down bread from Heaven (Exodus 16:4) and provided His people with food. Jesus reminds them that the Lord is their ultimate Provider, and they do not have to worry about anything if they put their full trust in Him (Matthew 6:26). As the Lord provided the ancient Israelites with physical food, He was providing (and still provides) His people with spiritual food in Jesus.

Jesus admonishes the crowd for their rejecting of this essential spiritual food (John 6:36-37). Although they could see Him, they did not believe Him. The gospel is summarized again for them by Jesus. He foretells of His death, burial, and resurrection and tells them that if they accept Him as the Bread of Life, they will also have eternal life (John 6:38-40). These realities are true for us today and will forever be true! After hearing this, the Jewish leaders showed their hardened hearts by grumbling and rejecting Him (John 6:41-42). Jesus reminds us that He has to reveal Himself to us for us to be able to believe (John 6:44-47). If you are unsure that Jesus has revealed Himself to you, pray. Ask Him to make it abundantly clear that He is revealing Himself to you so that you can accept Him as the Bread of *your* life. If this is bringing to mind a loved one who may not be accepting the Bread of Life, pray for them. When you think you have prayed too much, pray again! Jesus wants everyone to come to Him and accept Him as King (1 Timothy 2:3-4). We can never pray too much for God to reveal Himself to our hearts or the hearts of others.

Anyone who eats literal bread (or any food) will eventually physically die because of sin. If we accept Jesus as the Bread of Life, while our earthly bodies will still die, our souls find eternal life in Jesus (John 6:50-51). If we do not accept this Bread of Life, we have no true life in us (John 6:53-58). Jesus is our life and our everything from the moment we first accept Him as our Savior, and we can have the assurance of salvation in Him. This is more important than any physical food.

Jesus does, however, value physical food and recognize our need for it. If He did not, He would not use bread as a comparison to Himself. As we establish that Jesus is more important, we can begin to understand what Jesus says about food and how to fuel and nourish our earthly bodies.

More than Jesus cares about food, He cares more about our hearts. Contrary to diet culture beliefs, the types and amounts of food that you choose to eat or not eat do not define you. Jesus declared all foods clean in Mark 7:14-23 by stating that nothing outside of us (in this context, food) can defile us. In the Old Testament, God was very specific about which foods were clean and unclean. This had nothing to do with health and everything to do with approaching God in the right standing. God chose the Israelites as His people to be set apart. One of the ways that they were set apart, or different from the surrounding nations, was that they were able to approach their Creator. In order to approach God, they had to be clean. If they ate any food that God declared unclean, they could not approach God. Being clean in order to approach God included non-food-related things as well. Touching a dead body, for example, also makes someone unclean. Unclean simply meant that it was unfit to be used for the worship of God.[1] Jesus came to fulfill the Law, once and for all. Because of Jesus and His sacrifice, we no longer have to strive to be clean to approach God. Again, clean does not have anything to do with health.

In Biblical times, there was no such thing as a nutrition label. There was no way to know the number of calories or the macronutrient breakdown of any specific foods. All the people knew was that they needed food to fuel their bodies and survive. God did care about how people chose to eat, but he never instructed people to limit or eliminate any specific foods or food groups for sole health or wellness reasons. Now that we have the common grace of Western medicine and sound nutrition, we can follow guidance and medical nutrition therapy for certain health conditions, but there is no reason to add morality to foods or cut them out for the sake of being "better."

One argument against this can be found in the Daniel Plan (this is not to be confused with the Daniel Fast, based on Daniel 10. More on this later). The Daniel Plan was created by pastor Rick Warren and Dr. Oz, as well as two other physicians (note: not dietitians).[2] The plan is based on the book of Daniel and how Daniel and his friends' obedience to God led to better health. During the Babylonian exile, Daniel and his friends were in King Nebuchadnezzar's court, where they were offered the finest foods. They could not be sure, however, that these foods were kosher (or clean, according to God's definition). Because this was before Jesus came to fulfill the Law, they were still bound by the dietary restrictions that God put in place in Leviticus 11 and Deuteronomy 14.

They were not to eat a calf that could have been cooked in its mother's milk (no cheeseburgers or the mixing of any meat and dairy), as well as other types of animals that the Lord declared unclean (remember that unclean here does not mean "unhealthy"). Since Daniel and his friends were Jewish and wanted to honor God with how they ate, they likely abstained from eating all of the meat in Nebuchadnezzar's court while under his three-year training program. The chief was worried that the king would be offended that they would not eat the royal food and that their health would decline. This is where the "ten-day test" is recorded in Daniel 1:12. Daniel wanted to show the chief that he could follow the kosher diet, and thus obey God, while in this training. God does not command his people to intentionally do anything harmful to themselves, so sure enough, Daniel 1:15 said that after the ten-day test, they were "better in appearance" than the others who ate the king's food. They were stronger and their physical health was flourishing because they were following God's commands. Verse 15 continues to say that they were also "fatter" than the others. The Daniel plan conveniently overlooks this, likely because now we consider "fatness" to be synonymous with being unhealthy. During this time, fatness was actually considered more favorable because it meant that you could afford food and did not have to work with your hands.[3] This is an example of how beauty standards have changed, yet diet culture takes scripture out of context to justify restrictive dieting. The Daniel Plan is just another diet with a Christian label slapped on it. This diet advises following the same restrictive eating patterns that Daniel and his friends followed (out of necessity for obeying God). It claims that this is for "health reasons" rather than following God's commands because of what Jesus clearly states about food in Mark 7:15, as well as the knowledge that Christ came to fulfill the Law. Mark 7:15 states that *"nothing outside a person that by going into him can defile him, but the things that come out of a person are what defile him."* Mark 7:19 goes on to explicitly say that Jesus *"declared all foods clean."*

The Daniel Fast is another plan glorified by the diet industry that is based on reading Daniel 10 through the lens of diet culture. For more on what this fast is and what it entails, see chapter 12 of this book. Different sources have different recommendations, but the bottom line is that it is a restrictive (usually a semi-vegan) diet and not an actual fast. Fasting is not about "improving physical health." If this is the intent, it is no longer a spiritual fast, but a diet.

God does care about how we eat and how we treat our bodies, so we are to steward our bodies well; however, stewarding our bodies does not mean strictly monitoring what we eat and constantly pursuing body change. We are to eat in a way that feels good, honors our body's specific needs, and enjoys God's good creation. We should listen to our God-given hunger signals unless there is a specific medical reason not to (early stages of eating disorder recovery being one example). God created us with intention, and we should treat our bodies with kindness and respect.

. . .

PRAYER

Dear God,

Thank you for all that You say about food in the Bible. Forgive me for the ways that I have prioritized what the world says about food over what You say. Help me to view food as a good gift and to see Jesus as the true bread of life and all that I truly need.

In Jesus' name, amen.

SOURCES:

1. "What does the Bible mean when it says something is unclean?" GotQuestions.org. https://www.gotquestions.org/Bible-unclean.html

2. Warren R. The Daniel Plan : 40 Days to a Healthier Life. Grand Rapids: Zondervan Books; 2020.

3. Eknoyan G. A history of obesity, or how what was good became ugly and then bad. *Adv Chronic Kidney Dis.* 2006;13(4):421-427. doi:10.1053/j.ackd.2006.07.002

4. "What is a Daniel Fast?" GotQuestions.org. https://www.gotquestions.org/Daniel-fast.html. Accessed May 23, 2024.

10

SOUND NUTRITION

Intuitive Eating, Nutritional Science, and Gentle Nutrition

*"And God said, "Behold, I have given you every plant yielding
seed that is on the face of all the earth, and every tree with seed
in its fruit. You shall have them for food."*
~ Genesis 1:29 (ESV)

AS A DIETITIAN (and a future dietitian), we would be doing all our readers a disservice if we did not spend some time talking about food and nutrition, including the basic principles of gentle nutrition. The original Intuitive Eating book is based on 10 principles of improving your relationship with food. Intuitive eating can be briefly described as listening to your body, eating what you want when you want, and honoring your internal hunger and fullness cues while rejecting diet culture beliefs.ᴬ Authors Evelyn Tribole and Elyse Resch explain that gentle nutrition is the tenth and final principle of intuitive eating for a reason: it is essential to heal your relationship with food and your body first, and *then* you can begin to implement nutrition facts into your food choices from a place of self-care rather than fear.[1] While the Intuitive Eating book is an excellent resource, it is a secular resource that does not include the importance of letting Jesus into your healing process. If you feel like you are in a good place with food and body image, but Jesus feels far away and out of the body image picture, please consider whether reading this chapter would be beneficial for you right now (1 Corinthians 6:12) and feel the freedom to skip it if needed. Gentle nutrition can be defined as using the information that you know about nutrition to make informed food choices from a place of freedom and self-care.

Believe it or not, nutritional knowledge can be your friend, not just your one-way ticket to guilt and shame. With this in mind, let us dive into the science of food! All foods are made up of macronutrients and micronutrients. Macronutrients are carbohydrates, proteins, and fats. Micronutrients are vitamins and minerals. Micronutrients are great, but if you are not getting enough macronutrients, you are not going to absorb all of the vitamins and minerals (micronutrients) you are consuming. It is more important to ensure that you are eating enough than to over-prioritize vitamins and minerals.

Carbohydrates are made up of sugar. Sugar is not bad. It is essential. There are several different types of sugar molecules, including: glucose (a single molecule), sucrose, lactose, and maltose (two sugar molecules), and fructose and sucrose (multiple sugar molecules). When you eat a carb (any carb), the sugar molecules go into the bloodstream, and they are *all* converted into glucose (the simplest form of sugar) in the liver. Thus, saying you are "eating no sugar" is impossible. When your cells realize that you have glucose in the bloodstream, the pancreas releases insulin. Insulin does many things in the body, but one function is that it opens up our cells so that glucose can go in and get turned into energy (in the form of ATP). Our brain predominately runs on glucose, and our red blood cells run off of glucose only. If you are starving to death, your body will have no more available glucose to use for energy, and your brain will switch to using ketones. This is not favorable and should be avoided if possible due to the strain that it puts on your other organs, specifically the liver and kidneys. All of our organs, besides the brain, are glucose-sparing, which means that they can run off of other forms of energy (such as amino acids from protein) in times of need. Because our brains need a consistent and steady supply of glucose, it is important to eat some form of carbohydrate at every meal and snack.

The recommended dietary allowance (RDA) for all Americans is that ~45-65% of your daily energy should come from carbs. This amount is even higher for special populations, such as athletes. This is about half of your plate for any given meal. The diet culture idea that half of your plate should be non-starchy vegetables is not backed by sound nutritional biochemistry. Vegetables are great, but again, if you do not consume enough carbs, proteins, and fats, you will not absorb all of the nutrients in the veggies. Some examples of carbs include both whole grain and white pasta, rice, cereal, bread, chips, crackers, baked goods, fruits, and starchy vegetables, such as potatoes, beans, peas, and corn.

While all carbohydrates do the same thing in the body (give your brain and other organs the energy needed to function properly), there is a slight difference between high-fiber and low-fiber carbohydrates. Higher fiber carbohydrates include whole grains, fruits, and vegetables. It is important to note that when comparing two very similar foods where the only difference is the fiber content (for example, one slice of white bread vs. the same size slice of whole grain bread), the total amount of glucose is roughly the same. They both give your brain the same amount of energy. The difference is the amount of time it takes for your cells to metabolize that energy. The white carb gives quicker energy, whereas the whole grain carb is slower and more sustained. This relates to fiber. Diet culture would like you to believe that you should always only choose the high-fiber option.

However, it always depends on the need. If you are on your way out of the door for a quick walk or jog, the white carb would be the better option because it gives you the quickest energy. If you are finishing out your workday and know it will be a few hours before your next meal or snack, the whole grain, higher fiber option may be better to keep you full for longer and have more "staying power." If you are in eating disorder recovery and experiencing gastroparesis or delayed gastric emptying/slowed digestion (which is very common), the white carb is actually better because it is digested more quickly and can prepare you better for your next meal or snack on your meal plan.

Essentially, fiber is a unique type of carbohydrate that cannot be broken down into sugar molecules to be digested. Fiber, therefore, feeds your gut microbes to promote a flourishing gastrointestinal tract, but because it cannot be digested, it is possible to have too much fiber. Excessive fiber intake can exacerbate bloating, gas, abdominal cramping, constipation, and nausea. It can also cause dehydration (since fiber pulls water in to dilute), decreased overall nutrient intake (from increased satiety due to intestinal bulk), and decreased absorption of some minerals (because insoluble fiber will decrease the time food has to interact with the GI tract for this absorption). Therefore, fiber is not the "end all be all." Two types of fiber are soluble and insoluble fiber. Insoluble fiber will increase the bulk in your intestines to speed up digestion speed. Soluble fiber, on the other hand, will slow down the digestion rate. There are benefits when we eat enough fiber, but this should not be prioritized over all of your body's other essential food needs.

Proteins, another macronutrient, are the building blocks of cells, and they are made up of amino acids. Protein may be the only macronutrient that has not been demonized by diet culture in the last decade. Protein is involved in muscle and tissue growth and repair, immunity, and pH balance, among many other functions. Proteins make up enzymes and some hormones. Proteins have the same amount of energy as carbs but are more difficult for our cells to digest. Therefore, proteins have more "staying power," meaning they keep you full for longer. Eating a combination of both carbs and protein can fill you up for longer than just carbs or proteins on their own. Because we know the essentiality of glucose (carbohydrates) and our cell's tendency to be glucose-sparing, proteins cannot play their role in building muscle unless there is adequate carbohydrate in the diet. This is because if you are not eating enough carbohydrates, your body will break down your muscles to convert amino acids to glucose in a process called gluconeogenesis so that your body (especially your brain) has the fuel that it needs to function.

There are twenty total amino acids that your body needs to function properly, eleven of which your body can create (non-essential amino acids), and nine of which you must consume in the diet (essential amino acids). Animal proteins contain all nine essential amino acids. They are complete proteins. Quinoa and soy are also complete proteins. If you choose to eat a plant-based diet, you can get all the necessary amino acids; it just requires more thought and intentionality. There may be ethical reasons, or even occasional medical nutrition reasons, that someone chooses to or is advised to eat a plant-based diet, but there is no conclusive evidence that shows eating plant-based is objectively "healthier."

If you find yourself following a plant-based diet for "health reasons," spend some time in prayer and examine if this may be another disordered food rule. It may also be helpful to meet with a Registered Dietitian to discuss this further and learn more about your specific needs. If you are following a plant-based diet, or even enjoying a meatless meal, four non-animal-based foods contain several essential amino acids (but not all nine): nuts/seeds, dairy, whole grains, and legumes. As long as a meal or snack has two of these four foods, all 9 essential amino acids are covered. This is called complementing proteins. Some examples of plant-based options with complete proteins are a peanut butter sandwich, cheese cubes and mixed nuts, rice and beans, and yogurt with granola.

Once again, having protein and a carb together increases satiety in meals and snacks. It is recommended that ~15-25% of your total daily energy intake should come from protein. This is roughly ¼ of your plate if you are eating animal protein. If you choose to eat only plant-based protein, the total volume of food will be greater because most of your carbohydrates are also a source of protein. If there is no animal protein on the plate, it is recommended to double the carb/starch portion (one serving is your carb, and one serving is your protein on the plate).

Last but certainly not least is fats. Fats have the most "staying power" of all of the macronutrients in terms of how much energy they supply. Because of this, the standard serving size is the smallest. In other words, you would not eat the same volume of olive oil as you would of rice. Nonetheless, fat is essential for long-term satiety and plays a part in supporting vital organs, generating body heat to keep you warm, maintaining the health and strength of hair, skin, and nails, and providing energy storage in times of need, to name a few. If you have been eating a low-fat diet and start to reintroduce fats, you may notice that your hair looks shinier and thicker, you do not feel as cold all the time, and you have more energy throughout your day. This is because fat is doing its job in your body!

Fat also improves and enhances the flavor, texture, and aroma of foods. Fat-soluble vitamins (vitamins A, D, E, and K) cannot be digested without fat. Thus, if you make a salad with all of the colors of the rainbow (lots of micronutrients) but put a fat-free dressing on it, your body will not absorb all of the vitamins and minerals on your plate. Fat is responsible for your brain's structural communication network (which is why infants, after one year of age, are instructed to drink whole milk over low to no-fat milk). It is also an important regulator and component of hormones, such as cholesterol, for cell membrane fluidity and sex hormones. Interestingly, fat may also impact the status of our mental health. Studies show that a low-fat diet is associated with increased levels of depression.[2] This makes sense for two reasons: 1) Fat is responsible for the structural communication network of the brain, and 2) Fat makes food taste good, so eating bland and non-enjoyable food certainly cannot help with mental health. Examples of fats include butter, all cooking oils, such as olive, vegetable, and canola oil, salad dressings, avocados, nuts/seeds, and dairy.

There are two types of fats: saturated and unsaturated fats. Both fats function in all the ways mentioned above. It is recommended that most fats be unsaturated (this includes oils that are liquid at room temperature and avocados). Unsaturated fats have at least one double bond in the hydrocarbon chain, which causes a "kink" and makes these fats unable to stack together as tightly. Because of this biochemistry and the fact that not all carbons have hydrogens attached, they are more easily digested and broken down. While it is recommended to consume mostly unsaturated fats, it is more important to ensure that you are getting enough fat than to police the specific types of fat that you are eating. It is better to have saturated fats than no fats at all.

In taking into account what is enjoyable, you will probably have a mix of both types of fats, so if it feels tasty, put the butter on your toast and sauté your veggies in olive oil (and, of course, if you prefer to do it differently, listen to your body and your preferences). The RDA for fat is ~25-35% of your total daily energy intake. Because fat is more energy-dense, this is a much smaller amount on the plate. This could be sauteing your vegetables in oil, having a dinner roll with butter, and the fat in your meat that is ¼ of the plate.

The bottom line is that labeling foods as "good/bad" or "healthy/unhealthy" is unhelpful and only keeps you stuck in food guilt. Remember, you should never feel guilty for what you are eating unless there was sin involved (for example, if you stole the food). It is more helpful to think about food in the ways that the Lord made it: to provide nutrients for our bodies' survival, flourishing, and enjoyment, and to receive it with a grateful heart. All foods can have a place in a balanced diet. When we shift our focus from what is "bad" about certain foods to what they can provide for us, we can begin to view food from a place of joy. Every single food can provide you with one of these essential things: carbohydrates, proteins, fats, micronutrients, and pleasure (yes, pleasure is good and right; see Ecclesiastes 9:7). Giving yourself unconditional permission to eat means allowing yourself to eat certain foods just because they bring your taste buds pleasure. After all, the Lord blessed us by giving us tasty food. We can bring Him worship and honor by enjoying our food.

. . .

PRAYER

Dear Jesus,

You are the bread of life! You are so good! Help me to remember that You are all that I need. When I have thoughts about changing my body or when I see the foods that I eat as something I should feel guilty for, it reminds me of what my body needs. You are the most important thing. I want to see food as a good gift, but You as the most important thing in my life. Help me to fix my gaze upon you.

In Your name, amen.

11

GLUTTONY

"It is not what goes into the mouth that defiles a person, but what comes out of the mouth; this defiles a person."
~ Matthew 15:11 (ESV)

WHAT IS GLUTTONY? If there is freedom in Christ, even with food and body image, how do we accept gluttony as a sin? Is overeating a sin? What about binge eating? These words do not all mean the same thing. The aim of this chapter is to understand what these words mean without the lens of diet culture. Gluttony is, without a doubt, a sin, but we need to have a better understanding of what gluttony really is (and is not).

Overeating is often lumped in with gluttony, as though they are synonyms, but this is not always the case. Let us first define overeating. Overeating means eating more than your body's needs. It is eating past comfortable fullness and ignoring your body's internal hunger/fullness signals. If you are in eating disorder recovery and under the care of a treatment team, including a dietitian, eating past comfortable fullness will likely be a part of your recovery because this is restoring your body to a place that is free from the disorder. This is a normal part of eating disorder treatment and is not bad.

Sometimes, overeating is a part of normal eating. For example, let us say it is your birthday, and you want to enjoy a nice steak at your favorite steakhouse. You do not eat that meal every day, possibly because of the cost or because of convenience. You are almost certainly going to want to eat past comfortable fullness because you are celebrating. Then, just as you are feeling a little too full, the server brings out a slice of cake and sings Happy Birthday. At the end of the night, you probably feel a little physically uncomfortable. While this could be considered overeating, it is definitely normal, given the circumstances. In general, this kind of overeating is not an issue because feeling physically uncomfortable is not a pleasant experience.

Additionally, the Bible addresses feasting very specifically and often associates it with gladness and celebration (Esther 9). The celebration surrounding meals honors God and cultivates the community. This also cultivates gratitude and worship. Even Jesus' first miracle was around a wedding feast in John 2:1-12! Because feasting is addressed so often in scripture, chapter 13 is dedicated to this topic.

On the other hand, joy and celebration, though overeating, can be done repeatedly in response to dieting. This is normalized by the phrases "cheat days" and "starting over tomorrow." This is also seen through "cut and bulk season" and binges. People may overeat in response to not trusting in God's provision for them that there will be enough food to eat later, especially those who experience food insecurity or have in the past. Another common reason people overeat is to drown out challenging feelings and emotions. Eating can be a way to cope with feelings (imagine when you were a child getting ice cream if you had a bad day at school or turning to sweets after a breakup as a teen or adult). This can become an issue if food is your only coping mechanism. Proverbs 25:16 also makes a clear warning about overeating and says, *"If you find honey, eat just enough— too much of it, and you will vomit."* This does caution us of our body's biological response to too much of a good thing. This wisdom proverb instructs us to eat enough to satisfy our hunger but not to consistently overeat and make ourselves sick.

Second, let us define binge eating. According to the Diagnostic and Statistical Manual of Mental Disorders, 5th edition (DSM-5), binge eating is characterized by at least three of the following: eating more rapidly than normal, eating until feeling uncomfortably full, eating large amounts of food when not physically hungry, eating alone due to embarrassment, and/or feeling disgusted, depressed, or very guilty after overeating.[1] Unless someone's binge episodes are recurrent and persistent in nature, this is not a binge eating disorder. Binge eating *can, of course,* be gluttony, but often there is more going on. Unlike the lies that diet culture tells you, food itself is often not the issue when it comes to binge eating disorder recovery but the condition of the heart. Eating disorder recovery is complex and highly individualized. If you struggle with overeating that feels compulsive, or if you struggle with a binge eating disorder, there is freedom here, too. Full recovery is possible without the shame and guilt of bondage to sin because we are no longer slaves to sin!

Finally, let us define gluttony. "Glutton" or "gluttony" appears in the Bible six times, four times in the Old Testament and twice in the New Testament.[A] As often as the word "glutton" creeps into the church, it is surprising that gluttony is mentioned so few times in scripture. As one of the "seven deadly sins," one would think that the Bible speaks more specifically and directly to this sin.[B] The truth is that every sin is deadly, but the sin of gluttony is often elevated because of diet culture. People emphasize what they care about, yet God calls sin, sin.

The Hebrew word for glutton is *zálal*, and it means "to be worthless or lavish, a squanderer; to make light of."[2] The first use of *zálal* in the Bible is Deuteronomy 21. This passage discusses what to do if a young man (not speaking of a child) is disobeying the fifth commandment by not honoring his father and mother (Deuteronomy 5:16). Deuteronomy 21:20 states to announce to the city, *"This our son is stubborn and rebellious; he will not obey our voice; he is a glutton and a drunkard."* Verse 21 goes on to command stoning him to death for his sin if found guilty. In this context, *zálal* refers to the young boy as a squanderer. The issue here is a man's deviant behavior (wrong heart posture), not the food he is eating. The son has persistent dominating urges and appetites against the Lord's command to obey his parents. In Proverbs 28:7, a *"companion of gluttons"* is referred to as shameful to the family. This argument, once again, is about a wrong heart posture toward the Law. This is followed by verse 8, which states, "whoever multiplies his wealth by interest and profit..." If indulgence in food is *continually and unnecessarily* wasting one's resources for selfish desires, then this is gluttony.

Another example of where gluttony has nothing to do with food is found in Titus 1:12. This section of Titus discusses the qualifications for elders in the church and, therefore, is more concerned about the vitality of the church body if the Cretens were left to themselves. These people were not to see food and drink as what satisfies them, for food can only satisfy their belly. But the Lord alone satisfies their soul. Food is a gift, but it perishes!!

Only once is zálal used in regard to food. Proverbs 23:20-21 gives the following advice: "Be not among drunkards or among gluttonous eaters of meat, for the drunkard and the glutton will come to poverty, and slumber will clothe them with rags." The entire book of Proverbs contrasts wisdom and folly. In this context, this means "to be a lavish or worthless eater of meat." This is a warning to not associate with people who have given in to and are at peace with lustful living. Again, while food is the tool used to sin, the sin here is the unruly heart posture. CS Lewis discusses in The Screwtape Letters how the problem with gluttony is paying too much attention to food, and not the food itself.[3]

When studying scripture, it is important to look at the entire chapter to gain important information about the context and the bigger picture. In Proverbs 23:1, we are given the warning that when you sit down to eat with a rich ruler, you need to be aware of the situation. Verse 2 goes on to instruct us to "put a knife to [our] throat[s] if [we] are given to appetite." This is a warning against sensuality. The rich host here is using his luxuries to entrap his guests to do his bidding for him. He buys them nice food to take advantage of them. The warning here is to be sober-minded and not be easily won over by expensive luxuries. A modern-day example would be Libby going on a first date with a young man she met on a dating app, Joey. Joey takes Libby out to a nice dinner, and at the end of the night, pays for the check, making it very clear that he is expecting something from Libby in return. Joey is paying for Libby's dinner to put Libby in his debt, so she feels obligated to "return the favor" later on in the night. This scenario is what Proverbs 23 warns about. The wise thing for Libby to do would be to pay for her own dinner and leave or just decide to go home alone after dinner.

In the New Testament, the Greek word for glutton is *phagos,* which means "to devour or consume; to take food."[4] This is a little more in line with how diet culture defines "gluttony," but it still does not hit the nail on the head. When discussing the messengers from John the Baptist, Jesus describes the criticism that both He and John received:

"For John came neither eating nor drinking, and they say, 'He has a demon.' The Son of Man came eating and drinking, and they say, 'Look at him! A glutton and a drunkard, a friend of tax collectors and sinners!' Yet wisdom is justified by her deeds." (Matthew 11:18-19)

The people criticized Jesus for eating and drinking. The people of ancient Jerusalem had an understanding of *phagos,* and because Jesus was not the king and conqueror coming in on a throne with a white horse, they criticized him, calling him a glutton. We know that Jesus was the only person who ever lived without sin, so this inaccurate assessment of Him was intended to be an insult. The parallel passage in Luke 7:34 also uses *phagos* to describe what people were saying about our Savior. Again, when we revisit the word *zálal,* this was their understanding of gluttony. They were accusing

Jesus (falsely) of having a lavish and squandering heart posture toward food.

Additionally, four of the six times gluttony appears in the Bible, it shows up with the word drunkard (Deuteronomy 21:20, Proverbs 23:20-21, Matthew 11:13, and Luke 7:34). There is a sense of unruly extravagance, laziness, and disobedience that comes along with the heart posture of a glutton. This makes sense when you consider what sets eating and gluttony apart, as well as drinking and drunkenness apart. Drinking alcohol is not a sin. In fact, scripture states in Psalm 104:15 that wine *"gladden[s] the heart of man."* The point is that consuming alcohol is not sinful, but drinking to the point of drunkenness is. Drunkenness in itself is a response to what is going on in the heart.

In the same way, eating is not a sin (Matthew 15:11), but eating in a lavish and squandering way is. The root of both sins is the condition of the heart. To help illustrate the heart condition in question, let us take a look at another modern-day example.

Laura was a hard-working wife and mother of four children ages 10-18. Laura tried every diet in the book when it came to losing her "baby weight" after her fourth child. She was on and off diets for several years. After her final attempt at lasting weight loss, she threw in the towel and decided to give up. Since she could not sustainably lose weight, she decided to eat "whatever, whenever." She would leave work in the afternoon to pick her kids up from school, go through the drive-through, order a meal, and finish it before she made it to school. She would eat a snack with her children after school, and then, despite not being physically hungry, she would often get seconds of dinner that she prepared for her family. While this pattern did not happen every day, it was always in response to her frustration that she could not lose weight. Sometimes, after her family was asleep, she would go to the refrigerator and have an additional snack despite not being hungry. Before this habit started, Laura would spend her evening hours alone in her personal quiet time reading scripture and praying to God with a grateful heart. Since her frustration around her lack of body change started, her heart was set on her body, and she was actively ignoring the Holy Spirit in her life (Colossians 3:2). When she talked to her friends from her Bible study, they acknowledged that this was a sin, but advised her to "just try harder and stop eating so much." Instead of asking her about the condition of her heart, they gave the unhelpful advice to simply stop sinning (attempts to behavioral modification over heart transformation). When she eventually sought professional help, she could not remember the last time she personally prayed to the Lord outside of a family or group context, giving thanks for her meals, or even thanking him for the blessings that He had provided for her family. She had fallen into gluttony as a way of turning away from God. Once her heart posture was addressed, she could finally begin to address the behaviors.

Behavior change without heart change is never lasting, but if we are in Christ, we are not under the power of sin but under grace (Romans 6:14). Where sin abounds, grace abounds all the more. Gluttony is more complex than the one-off times of overeating. If you are stuck in the seemingly endless cycle of sin and gluttony, there is grace for you! God is rich in mercy. You do not have to live in bondage because we are saved by His grace (Ephesians 2:1-10). Walking in His grace means repenting of sin and turning toward Jesus as our helper.

We must ask ourselves: are we being wise and going to the Lord with all of our burdens, or are we turning to food and overeating as a band-aid to fix the burdens of our souls? If your heart is postured toward squandering or indulging in food, the food itself is not a sin. The way we eat *can be* sinful, but it is, first and foremost, the product of a sinful and broken heart. Where the world would say to feel guilty and "just try harder to eat less," your own best efforts cannot change your heart. Only God can do that (Jeremiah 20:12) through His Son, Jesus Christ (Acts 15:8). To be abundantly clear here: gluttony is a sin, *and* there is freedom in Christ to eat. When eating becomes a sinful coping mechanism or a tool to ignore the Holy Spirit in your life, there is grace and forgiveness in Christ, and healing is possible. As mentioned previously, Romans 6:1-2 says, *"Are we to continue in sin that grace may abound? By no means! How can we who died to sin still live in it?"* By turning from our sin and toward our loving Father (repentance), we can live in the fullness of His grace again and again.

. . .

PRAYER

Dear God,

Thank You for the ways that scripture is clear about gluttony. You are a good and forgiving Father. Because of You, I no longer have to walk in the bondage of sin. I confess where my heart posture may be wrong. Help me to see what it is like to honor You with my eating and drinking and not let my heart be placed on things that are not from You. Remove distractions that may be getting in the way of me living abundantly in your grace and mercy.

In Jesus' name, amen.

FOOTNOTES:

A. Upon a Blue Letter Bible search of "gluttony" and "glutton," these numbers were provided. Blue Letter Bible is an online concordance for finding where specific words or topics are used in the Bible. For more information on the Blue Letter Bible, please visit blueletterbible.org.

B. The "seven deadly sins" are part of Catholic tradition and are not explicitly listed in scripture. This is mentioned here as a reference to how some Churches can overemphasize something that is not as present in the Bible as the culture would lead us to believe.

SOURCES:

1. Diagnostic and Statistical Manual of Mental Disorders: DSM-5. 5th ed., American Psychiatric Association, 2013. DSM-V, doi-org.db29.linccweb.org/10.1176/appi.books.9780890425596.dsm02.

2. H2151 - zālal - Strong's Hebrew Lexicon (KJV). Blue Letter Bible. Accessed November 14, 2022. https://www.blueletterbible.org/lexicon/h2151/kjv/wlc/0-1/

3. Lewis CS. *The Screwtape Letters*. HarborOne; February 6, 2001.

4. G5314 - phagos - Strong's Greek Lexicon (KJV). Blue Letter Bible. Accessed November 15, 2022. https://www.blueletterbible.org/lexicon/g5314/kjv/tr/0-1/

1 2

FASTING

"But seek first the kingdom of God and his righteousness, and all these things will be added to you."
~ Matthew 6:33 (ESV)

FASTING IS AN overlooked spiritual discipline in the modern world that has many mixed messages around it, the main contributor being diet culture's emphasis on the pursuit of intentional weight loss. One certain thing, though, is that fasting is important to God. In fact, it is mentioned over 70 times throughout the Bible.[A] As you observe Jesus' life, He fasted! In Luke 4, Jesus fasted *"for forty days, being tempted by the devil. And he ate nothing during those days. And when they ended, he was hungry."* If our whole life purpose is to conform more and more to the image of Christ (sanctification), then why wouldn't we also fast?

Let us break this down and look at places in scripture indicating we should fast. During the Sermon on the Mount, Jesus' most famous sermon, He says, "*When* you fast..." Notice that Jesus did not say if you fast but *when*.[1] Fasting is actually a command to us! Another example is Acts 14, which shows us the early church was committed to prayers and fasting. In Joel 2:12, believers are exhorted to return their hearts to the Lord with fasting. God does not need anything from us, but He *wants* our whole hearts and indicates this even further in Matthew 6:33 when Jesus tells us to seek first His Kingdom. Every kingdom we build for ourselves is in vain. In fasting, we receive the tangible reminder that God is the one sustaining us. We are reminded of our neediness for God as our source of life over any other thing this world has to offer. And our utter dependence gives Him more of our heart! During times that would be spent enjoying a meal, we spend time in prayer, communicating with our Father in Heaven.

We see the importance of fasting because Jesus fasted, but how does fasting practically help our minds focus more on God? Isaiah 58 is a chapter about fasting but begins with admonishment against fasting for their own desires and prosperity over obedience to God's commands. This resulted in fasting being an empty ritual rather than practicing the presence of God. God's people tried to amplify their own voice (Isaiah 58:4) rather than amplify worship to God. When we look at Jesus' life on earth, we see our Savior was filled with compassion. There are many times throughout scripture where Jesus reaches out to the needy. As we seek to follow in Jesus' example, fasting is an opportunity for our hard hearts to grow in compassion toward the poor and needy (Isaiah 58:6-7). It is a humbling experience to choose hunger for a short time while we have food available to reflect on those who have no choice.

Furthermore, rather than seeing fasting as a time to save money from a meal or two, our hearts can be grown toward sacrificial generosity.[1] How lovely is it to provide a meal to someone in need with the money that would have been used for ourselves (Proverbs 22:9, Isaiah 58:7). When love for God and others marks our lives (Matthew 22:36-38), the Lord works miraculous ways in our life (Isaiah 58:8-12). He knows what we need more than we know what we need, and He does not forsake the righteous (Psalm 37:25)! If you are feeling far from God, humble yourself before Him and fast.

Fasting can and should be done in the context of both community and in secrecy. Similar to the admonishment in the beginning of Isaiah 58, Matthew 6:16 commands, *"When you fast, do not look somber as the hypocrites do, for they disfigure their faces to show others they are fasting."* As Christ's followers, we live for an audience of one, and we boast in the Lord alone. We do not partake in spiritual disciplines to "check a box." 2 Timothy 3:5 also cautions against those who appear godly but deny God's power. In other words, people should not fast in order to look like a "better Christian." Fasting should be a practice between you and the Lord. Therefore, sometimes fasting in secrecy is a great way to grow your intimacy with Him. At other times, it is a good and Biblical discipline to gather your community together to seek the throne of God through prayer and fasting. Ezra 8:21-23 is a great example of this, where Ezra and his band of exiles seek God together for protection on their journey to Jerusalem. Moreover, Acts 13:2 and 14:23 are both examples of fasting within the context of a local church.

Fasting is also a way to resist the desires of our flesh. This is probably where diet culture takes fasting out of context the most. We know that hunger cues are God-given signals to us, and we need to eat to honor our bodies. Food is for survival, the flourishing of our physical bodies, and energy to live joyfully and serve God's kingdom. Our physical bodies have other appetites, like consumerism, power, sexual immorality, gossip, drunkenness, etc., that we often sinfully give into.[1] These lead to destruction and death (Romans 6:23). However, Galatians 5:22 states that self-control is a fruit of the Spirit that we are given once we believe in Jesus as our Lord and Savior.[B] Fasting is, therefore, a spiritual discipline to starve these destructive appetites of our flesh that draw us away from God.[1] Food, water, air, and shelter are needed for survival. Because food is a necessity to sustain life, when we fast from something essential to our bodies, we can be empowered in the Spirit to resist the fleshly desires of things that are not essential to our survival. The Apostle Paul even reminds us of this, exclaiming, *"But if we have food and clothing, with these we will be content"* (1 Timothy 6:8). He then contrasts these needs to a warning of our body's *"senseless and harmful desires that plunge people into ruin and destruction"* (1 Timothy 6:9).

Fasting shows us the sufficiency of Christ our King. Now, as a caveat, if someone is actively engaging in disordered eating behaviors, fasting from food may not be the best decision right now. In the Bible, we really do not see any examples of people "fasting" from anything other than food; however, 1 Corinthians 7:5 discusses self-control in the area of sexual immorality stating, *"Do not deprive each other except perhaps by mutual consent and for a time, so that you may devote yourselves to prayer. Then come together again so that Satan will not tempt you because of your lack of self-control."* This would be more of an example of abstinence, but abstinence can nonetheless grow our muscle for self-control.[B] An example of abstinence for someone engaging in disordered eating patterns could be abstaining from exercise. If exercise is a compulsive behavior to reach some ideal, not exercising is starving your fleshly desires while keeping your body healthy and safe. Other examples could be abstaining from social media, shopping, caffeine, or makeup.

Looking at specific fasts, we see this crossover of faith and diet culture with Lent. Lent is not about legalism but about remembering and honoring Christ. Lent should draw us into a closer relationship with God, but instead, Lent is often misused by diet culture. Oftentimes, people choose to cut out certain food groups for the forty days of Lent. Colossians 2:16-17 brings our gaze back to this, cautioning, *"Let no one judge you in food or in drink, or regarding a festival or a new moon or sabbaths, which are a shadow of the things to come, but the substance is of Christ."*

F.F. Bruce commented on this verse, saying, "It would be preposterous indeed for those who had reaped the benefit of Christ's victory to put themselves voluntarily under the control of the powers which he had conquered."[2] Jesus is the One who makes us clean, not cutting out certain food groups. The New Covenant of Jesus Christ declares food does not defile us. Instead, *"Everything created by God is good, and nothing is to be rejected if it is received with thanksgiving, for it is made holy by the word of God and prayer"* (1

Timothy 4:4). We know that God created food for us to eat (Genesis 1:29). If your faith community practices Lent, this is not to say you should not participate. Participate with your community, but consider giving something up that is not food-related if your intentions lean toward disordered eating and a "health" devotion over devotion to God.

Another similar example of selectively cutting out foods is in the book of Daniel when Daniel "mourned for three weeks. [He] ate no delicacies, no meat or wine entered [his] mouth, nor did [he] anoint himself at all, for the full three weeks" (Daniel 10:2-3). The popular 'Daniel Fast' comes from this Scripture and is when meat, dairy, alcohol, and other rich foods are avoided for twenty-one days. Though people today practice a 'Daniel Fast,' we see Daniel never actually called his period of mourning a fast.[3] Culture today calls this a 'partial fast,' but in scripture, we have no examples of a partial fast.[4] This would be a Biblical example of abstinence. The call to fast in scripture has always been not consuming food at all. Daniel humbled himself before God through an ascetic lifestyle, which was a way of disciplining himself to not rely on things that made his life more comfortable amidst his mourning.[c] A chapter prior, Daniel 9:3 actually tells us Daniel sought the Lord with prayer and fasting for the repentance of his people. Thus, it is indeed interesting that God mentions a legitimate fast in chapter 9 but does not use the word "fast" in Daniel 10:2-3. Overall, the authorial intent of Daniel 10 is not Daniel's diet but about a vision Daniel receives that is crucial to the prophecies in Daniel 11 and 12.

We have the freedom to see the way in which we turn to certain foods over God in times of discomfort and chose to abstain from certain food groups, but more often than not, our attention becomes hyper-focused on restrictions and rules rather than focusing more on God (the purpose of fasting) and His good gift of food to us. It becomes a problem when there is an overemphasis on food instead of prayer. John Mark Comer, in his ministry of Practicing the Way, discusses the essentiality of reflection on spiritual disciplines to get the most out of your practice.[1] As is customary in diet culture, scripture is taken out of context to justify restrictive eating with the goal of "health," not spiritual growth. Because cutting food groups out is popular in the Christian community among Lent and Daniel fasting, it is crucial to invite God in to search your heart's true intentions and desires (Psalm 139:23-24). Ask God for wisdom so that we do not have the appearance of godliness and deny its power (2 Timothy 3:5). It is crucial to re-ground ourselves around the message of fasting.

All in all, fasting is an incredible way to reconnect our soul and our body, and it was never intended to be a means of achieving a certain weight. In disordered eating and eating disorders, these lines often become blurred, so what a way to bring us back to our bodies' natural, God-given cues! These biological cues are gifts to us. However, for those in recovery, this may not apply because there may be an absence of hunger/fullness cues. If you are in recovery, make sure you discuss this with your treatment team before deciding to go on any fast. Spend time in prayer and consider starting with abstinence from something that is not food, as suggested earlier. The prayer is that fasting would be an opportunity for us to grow in our relationship and dependence on the Lord and to grow in gratitude toward the food we do have to nourish our bodies and souls.

PRAYER

Dear God,

Thank You for not needing me to follow set rules; rather, You want my heart. Holy Spirit, would You invite me more into the practice of fasting with wisdom, for I know all wisdom comes from above. My heart and flesh may fail, but You are my portion forever. Use the practice of fasting to show me my utter weakness apart from you. As I become slowly set free from the bondage of disordered eating, help me to not feel false guilt when I choose to fast from other things. Lead me, Jesus. I know You go before me in all things. Hear my prayers and grow my compassion for Your people. Also, give me the boldness to speak out against the ways fasts are falsely used by diet culture.

In Jesus' name, amen.

FOOTNOTES:

A. Upon a Blue Letter Bible search of "fast," "fasting," "feast," and "feasting," these numbers were provided. Blue Letter Bible is an online concordance for finding where specific words or topics are used in the Bible. For more information on the Blue Letter Bible, please visit blueletterbible.org.
B. For more on the fruit of the spirit of self-control, read chapter 14.
C. Through the common grace of science, we now know that grief affects our appetite through the bidirectional communicator of the vagus nerve between our brain and gut.

SOURCES:

1. Comer JM. The fasting practice. Practicing the Way. Accessed May 20, 2024. https://www.practicingtheway.org/fasting?gad_source =1.
2. Guzik, D. Colossians 2- Answering the Colossian Heresy (Applying Truth to Colossian heresy, quote by FF Bruce on verses 16-17, Enduring Word). https://enduringword.com/bible-commentary/colossians-2/. Published December 16, 2015.
3. Daniel Chapter 10. Enduring Word. Published December 26, 2015. https://enduringword.com/bible-commentary/daniel-10/
4. Food In God's Place. The Daniel Fast, Still Not Biblical Fasting. https://www.foodingodsplace.com/daniel-fast-still-not-biblical-fasting/. Published January 25, 2013. Accessed May 27, 2024.

13

FEASTING

"Therefore, let no one pass judgment on you in questions of food and drink, or with regard to a festival or a new moon or a Sabbath. These are a shadow of the things to come, but the substance belongs to Christ."
~Colossians 2:16-17 (ESV)

WHILE DIET CULTURE encourages us to restrict our food intake and deprive our bodies of what they need, the Bible actually discusses feasting more than it discusses fasting. The concept of feasting occurs about 149 times in 134 verses in the ESV.ᴬ This is not to say that one topic is more important than the other, but it is to say that as often as feasting is discussed, it is often overlooked.

Colossians 2:16-17 reminds us that Christ came to fulfill the Law, and this is why we no longer practice the feasts in the specific timeline outlined in the Old Testament; however, this does not mean that we shouldn't seek to understand the importance and principle of this part of the Law. If we do not understand the Old Testament Law, how can we practice gratitude for Jesus' sacrifice and fulfillment of it? In Romans 14:5-6, Paul tells us that because of Christ, we are free to feast or not feast based on our own personal convictions. Like with the discipline of fasting, feasting is not all about the food. It is about enjoying the abundance of God's kindness toward us in the community.[1] The purpose is to point us toward our Creator, not overindulgence. God has given us good gifts of tasty food and the body of believers around us![1]

While feasting may look different today than during Old Testament times, we can look at Leviticus 23 for specific feasts God appointed. The Sabbath was a weekly day of feasting (Leviticus 23:3). In a time when there was no electricity or running water, preparing a meal took a substantial amount of time. All bread had to be made from scratch, and there were no microwaves to quickly heat or reheat. Preparing a feast for the Sabbath (a day of rest) likely took a full day, yet God commanded His people to spend time the day before the Sabbath preparing the feast so that they could enjoy it and rest. They were also to celebrate the Passover (Leviticus 23:5). Just like Easter is a holiday to remind us of Jesus' resurrection from the dead, the Passover was a holiday to remind the Israelites of God passing over their homes and preserving their firstborn sons before Jesus' First Coming, as discussed in Exodus 11-12. God describes several more feasts in Leviticus 23, all of which include celebration. These are the Feast of First Fruits, the Feast of Weeks, the Feast of Trumpets, and the Feast of Booths. The Feast of First Fruits (Leviticus 23:9-14) was to celebrate the first harvest of barley for the year. The people recognized that God was the one in charge of the weather to allow for a harvest (Genesis 8:22), and through this feast, they took delight in God as the ultimate provider! Today, we know God has provided everything we need through Jesus, and 1 Corinthians 15:20 claims Jesus' resurrection as *"the first fruits of those who have fallen asleep."* Thus, we are reminded in our feasting of Christ's redemption and of His Second Coming.

Similarly, the Feast of Weeks (Leviticus 23:15-22) was to celebrate the first harvest of wheat for the year. The Feast of Trumpets (Leviticus 23:23-25) marked the end of the agricultural season. Lastly, the Feast of Booths (Leviticus 23:33-44) occurred after the harvest finished, and God's provision and protection were celebrated during the 40 years in the wilderness. In this time, God brought Israel out of the land of Egypt. Today, God has brought us out of our enslavement to sin. These are just the feasts outlined in Leviticus 23, and this is not exhaustive of all of the feasts outlined in the Old Testament.

In the New Testament, we also see several feasts. Jesus uses a wedding feast in Matthew 22:1-14 to describe our reliance on Him for our salvation. In the Story of the Prodigal Son, the father celebrates his son coming back with a feast. Luke 15:24 states, *"For this my son was dead, and is alive again; he was lost, and is found,"* and so they celebrated! These two parables that Jesus used show us that feasting is an appropriate way to respond to His call on our lives today. Enjoying food in the community and celebrating belonging to Jesus is good and right!

In the Hebrew, "feast" is the word *moedim*.[2] Moedim means "appointed beforehand." Knowing that God is everywhere all the time (omnipresent) and sovereign over everything, it should not surprise us that each of these Jewish feasts was appointed by God to align with the coming of Jesus.[2] Therefore, studying scriptural feasts can help you learn more about Jesus! As Colossians 2:16-17 makes clear that feasts are only a shadow of Christ, Galatians 4:9-11 additionally speaks to those that try to uphold religion through feasts to gain righteousness, saying, *"Now that you have come to know God, or rather to be known by God, how can you turn back again to the weak and worthless elementary principles of the world, whose slaves you want to be once more? You observe days and months and seasons and years! I am afraid I may have labored over you in vain."* The Bible tells us not to celebrate *"with the old leaven, the leaven of malice and evil, but with the unleavened bread of sincerity and truth"* (1 Corinthians 5:7-8). Moreover, Jesus says in John 14:6 that He is Truth!

Because of Christ's First Coming, feasting today looks a lot different than it did in the Old Testament. One of the most common practices of feasting in America is through a Thanksgiving feast. Though Thanksgiving is not found in the Bible, it is rooted in Christian history, especially when the Pilgrims first settled in America. Many had died during the pilgrimage, yet when their food supply became too low, an unexpected ship arrived with the provision of food.[3] Thus, they gave thanks to God, who ordained this provision for them, and this day became a holiday. They also gave thanks to God for the provision of land and religious freedom. These Pilgrims recognized God's provision for them not only in the physical but also the spiritual. Today, feasting may also look like a family Easter lunch or a birthday dinner with friends and family. In Ecclesiastes 3:12-13, King Solomon says, *"I perceived that there is nothing better for them than to be joyful and to do good as long as they live; also that everyone should eat and drink and take pleasure in all his toil—this is God's gift to man."* Thus, it is good to have some pleasure in meals. If God did not want us to have food for fuel, He could have chosen any other way to give us energy. He could have made us machines. However, in His intentionality, He gave us the taste buds, variety of foods, and creativity to enjoy food while also receiving fuel from it.

. . .

PRAYER

Dear God,

Thank You for sending Jesus to fulfill the Law! Forgive me for all the times that I have judged another believer based on their own convictions. Cultivate a sense of gratitude and celebration in my heart for You that is according to my convictions, whether that be to celebrate with feasting or not. Place in me a desire to study your Word more. Would this cause me to fall in love more with You, Jesus. You deserve praise and thanksgiving forevermore!

In Jesus' name, amen.

FOOTNOTES:

A. Upon a Blue Letter Bible search of "fast," "fasting," "feast," and "feasting," these numbers were provided. Blue Letter Bible is an online concordance for finding where specific words or topics are used in the Bible. For more information on the Blue Letter Bible, please visit blueletterbible.org.

SOURCES:

1. Mathis D. The Lost Art of Feasting. Desiring God. https://www.desiringgod.org/articles/the-lost-art-of-feasting. Published November 22, 2016. Accessed June 27, 2024.
2. "How did Jesus fulfill the meanings of the Jewish feasts?" GotQuestions.org. https://www.gotquestions.org/Jewish-feasts.html. Accessed July 10, 2024
3. "What should be the focus of Christians on Thanksgiving?" GotQuestions.org. https://www.gotquestions.org/thanksgiving-Christian.html. Accessed July 10, 2024

14

SELF-CONTROL

"For this very reason, make every effort to supplement your faith with virtue, and virtue with knowledge, and knowledge with self-control, and self-control with steadfastness, and steadfastness with godliness, and godliness with brotherly affection, and brotherly affection with love. For if these qualities are yours and are increasing, they keep you from being ineffective or unfruitful in the knowledge of our Lord Jesus Christ."
~ 2 Peter 1:5-8 (ESV)

SELF-CONTROL IS "restraint exercised over one's own impulses, emotions, or desires."[1] 2 Timothy 1:7 tells us that self-control is a gift from God, and we know that God gives good gifts (James 1:17). Proverbs 25:28 even tells us, "*A man without self-control is like a city broken into and left without walls.*" Therefore, self-control is actually a good thing! Because it is a gift from God, we must steward it well.

Biblical self-control *is not* restrictive dieting or excessive exercise.

2 Peter 1:5-8 shows us that faith is at the forefront of self-control. When self-control is mentioned as a fruit of the Spirit in Galatians 5:22-23, the preceding verses discuss how we must walk by the Spirit. Walking is an active action, not passive, but it also demonstrates the necessity of faith in our life because *"faith is the assurance of things hoped for, the conviction of things not seen"* (Hebrews 11:1). Philippians 3:9 highlights the necessity of faith as Paul shows us that righteousness is through our faith in Christ, not by our own doing. With that said, it is important to note that growth in the Christian life does not just happen, like a toddler does not just grow to be five feet tall overnight. It is a slow journey of daily acts of obedience, often through self-control, that accumulates to an overall life of self-discipline surrendered to the Father.

When someone has their mind set on obtaining something, they will do whatever it takes to get it. Both Philippians 3:14 and 1 Corinthians 9:24-27 speak to the effort people exert to try to win prizes; however, these prizes are perishable. They do not satisfy or fulfill us. As humans, we can set our minds on something whole-heartedly if it is something we truly desire. Matthew 6:21 reminds us that *"where your treasure is, there your heart will be also."* Knowing how scripture speaks of this, we must ask ourselves: do you put the same into pursuing godliness as you do in obtaining worldly prizes?

Self-control, as seen in 2 Peter 1:5-8, is for us to cultivate moral excellence.[2] Excellence is not synonymous with perfection, nor is it striving for recognition and pride. Even Paul explains that striving is not because he is perfect or for the purpose of obtaining perfection (Philippians 3:12). Rather, seeking excellence in what we do is to honor God (Colossians 3:23-24). In Philippians 3:12-21, Paul writes about straining toward the goal of walking in the way of Jesus all the days of our life with diligence. There are a few helpful principles we can take from this passage.

First, we should be reminded of who we are and who we belong to. We live to reflect Christ, not reflect the person across from us in the gym whose body we idolize. When we fix our eyes on others rather than the person of Jesus, we forget what is ahead (Philippians 3:13). We must renew our minds with the true prize here on earth: more of Jesus (Philippians 3:14). When we do, we are able to express thanks for the body He has given us as a gift instead of being preoccupied with comparison. Philippians 3:17 furthermore tells us to *"keep your eyes on those who walk according to the example you have in us."* Do not fix your eyes on those who are going to perpetuate negative body image (the models and bodybuilders, edited social media pictures, endless TikTok videos, and reality TV shows).

Second, it is important to remember that we do not know the people's stories when we look at their bodies. Take the example of envying or coveting someone's body across the gym. You do not know what their relationship with food or body image is! When you see pictures or videos of someone's life on social media, it can be tempting to compare the "behind the scenes" of your life to their "highlight reel."

Diet culture loves the idea of "using willpower" against normal physiological functions like hunger. Culture talks about willpower as strength from within, but Psalm 18:32 reminds us our strength comes from God alone. Biblical self-control is God as our source of strength because the Spirit empowers us. However, the church may even perpetuate this idea when discussing self-control as a means of managing behavior. Diet culture loves to tell us that we can control our hunger and fullness cues and the way we look if we try hard enough. The noise we hear from diet culture traps us in striving for unrealistic and unhealthy goals. Nevertheless, self-control is indeed a fruit of the Spirit (Galatians 5:22).

How do we make sense of expressing this fruit of the Spirit while remembering God is sovereign over all? How do we distinguish between self-control and a control heart idol? A heart set on control leads to it becoming an idol and is rooted in selfishness and wanting less of God and more of our fleshly desires. The natural desires of our flesh directly contradict the desires of the Spirit because of sin (Galatians 5:17). Exercising self-control is restraining yourself from engaging in your heart idol and instead surrendering this desire to the Lord.

A helpful way to think of self-control is boundaries that protect you.[2] Recall the heart idols discussed in chapter 6; at the root of every idol is the belief that something or someone can provide more than God. This is pride. However, in order to exercise self-control, humility is essential because you are confessing that destruction is inevitable if left to yourself. Only under this humility is someone able to recognize that self-control is actually a form of freedom rather than restraint. Another way scripture refers to the expression of self-control in our life is through being "sober-minded" (1 Peter 4:7).

What if demonstrating self-control was actually following a meal plan during eating disorder recovery even when everything in your mind does not want to? What if self-control is not engaging in old eating disorder behaviors, even though these behaviors seem comforting? What if it was deciding not to try "just one more diet" in an attempt to shrink your body? Our sin wants us to prioritize what is comfortable and routine, even if it is not serving us or our bodies well. Our hearts are filled with reckless, sinful desires, but we praise God for giving us the gift of the Holy Spirit who delights to help us exercise self-control.

. . .

PRAYER

Dear God,

Thank You for giving me the Holy Spirit as a helper to walk this earth. The heart is deceitful above all else, so would You help me not confuse a control heart idol for exercising self-control? I shall deny myself and take up my cross daily as You say in Luke 9:23. May self-control take me out of my comfort zone and grow me to look more like You, Jesus. Transform my heart to desire and help me to pursue godliness more than I pursue anything else here on earth, for everything else is fleeting.

In Jesus' name, amen.

S O U R C E S :

1. Self-control". Merriam-Webster.com Dictionary, https://www.merriam-webster.com/dictionary/self-control
2. Platt, D. Ever-Increasing Faith (2 Peter 1:5–7). Radical. https://radical.net/podcasts/pray-the-word/ever-increasing-faith-2-peter-15-7/. Published November 29, 2023. Accessed June 26, 2024.
3. Kim, J. To Be Free You Need Self-Control. The Gospel Coalition. https://www.thegospelcoalition.org/article/cultivate-free-life-self-control/. Published December 5, 2022. Accessed June 26, 2024

15

BODY IMAGE

Honoring God with Your Body

"Or do you not know that your body is a temple of the Holy Spirit within you, whom you have from God? You are not your own, for you were bought with a price. So glorify God in your body."
~ 1 Corinthians 6:19-20 (ESV)

PERHAPS THE MOST common verse taken out of context to justify restrictive dieting is 1 Corinthians 6:19-20. This verse is often used to claim that we should strive to look a certain way because our bodies are temples of the Holy Spirit, but when you look at this verse in context (all of 1 Corinthians 6:12-20), that is not what this verse refers to. The context of this verse is exhorting God's people to flee from sexual immorality. God is commanding us not to give away our bodies outside the covenant of marriage. Our bodies are indeed temples of the Holy Spirit, so we should honor God with our bodies. More on the implications for this in the context of marriage will be discussed in the next chapter, but it is important to note that this verse has nothing to do with dieting and exercising and everything to do with how we steward our sexuality.

When Paul wrote 1 Corinthians, he was writing to a culture that had a very skewed view of sex and sexuality. Sexual activity of all kinds was common in the Greek and Roman culture in Corinth. Because our current culture idolizes sex, too, there is a lot of worldly rationalization for sexual activity outside of the covenant of marriage. Paul wrote this passage to explain to the church in Corinth that how they express their sexuality matters. Yes, Jesus came to fulfill the Law, and the prohibitions on sex outside of marriage (like being "joined to a prostitute," 1 Corinthians 6:16) were still in place. At this time, it could be argued that Christ came to fulfill the Law. Therefore, the Christians of the time did not have to follow any of the restrictions God put in place in the Old Testament. While this is true, it is evident throughout the New Testament that even though ceremonial laws were fulfilled, moral laws were not nullified. For example, we still follow the 10 commandments (moral laws). This being said, God still cares about our hearts and how we express our sexuality. The point of 1 Corinthians 6:19-20 is not about dieting and exercising, so when we read these two verses alone without the context of the rest of 1 Corinthians 6, we are reading scripture through the lens of diet culture.

Besides honoring God's prescribed view of sex and sexuality

(Hebrews 13:4), what does it mean to glorify God in our bodies? Romans 12:1 urges us to *"present [our] bodies as a living sacrifice, holy and acceptable to God, which is [our] spiritual worship."* The ancient Israelites had to present a sacrifice to enter the presence of God. We no longer have to make sacrifices (thank you, Jesus!). Therefore, the way that we choose to listen to and honor our bodies is a form of spiritual worship. Stewarding our bodies well does not mean forcing them into restrictive diets or militant exercise. Remember, in chapter 6, we discussed that it *"is for freedom that Christ has set us free"* (Galatians 5:1). We steward the bodies that God gave us by eating in a way that is in tune with our bodies' needs. We walk in this freedom by giving ourselves permission to eat a variety of foods that contain carbohydrates, proteins, fats, and enjoyment. More on exactly how to eat in a way that glorifies God was covered in chapter 10. Good stewardship also means moving in a way that feels good and not forcing ourselves to exercise in a way that is worshiping the body rather than worshiping the Lord. Romans 12:2 goes on to remind us not to be *"conformed to this world, but [to] be transformed by the renewal of your mind, that by testing you may discern what the will of God is, what is good and acceptable and perfect."* Striving for a "perfect body" based on worldly standards is *"conforming to this world."*

In Philippians 1:20, Paul boldly states that Christ will be honored in his body, either by life or death. Philippians 1:21 says that *"to live is Christ, and to die is gain."* This is a reminder that our lives are not our own and that to live is to be here with Christ. As our lives are not our own, our bodies are not our own! 1 Corinthians 6:15 displays how becoming one with Jesus means you are inseparable from Him.

Scripture even refers to Jesus as the head of the body and His children as the body parts. In some way, our arms and legs are also Jesus' arms and legs! Though 1 Corinthians 6 does not justify diet culture, the passage nonetheless talks about the importance of our physical bodies. Therefore, when tempted to engage in disordered behavior, ask yourself, "Is this what Jesus wants for His body?"

Bodies do naturally change over time. The way someone looks when they are 10 is different when they are 20, which is also different from when they are 30, and so on. However, when we attempt to change or manipulate our bodies outside of their natural changes, we are deviating from God's perfect design. God created all bodies to be different. No two people are exactly the same, and that is intentional. When we fantasize about other's bodies or covet bodies that are not our own, this is sin (Exodus 20:17, Romans 7:7). Our bodies are the vessels that God graciously gave us to live in this life on earth to praise, please, and point to Him. Our society has objectified these vessels as "good" and "bad," but when God created humans in the garden, there was no dichotomy of good and bad bodies. Express thanks for how He has made you! This is an act of worship to King Jesus.

God said that creating the earth and all of the animals, land, birds, and everything that we see was good. However, God said that His humans were *"very good"* (Genesis 1:31) because He created us in His image. God's design for us is clearly unique, and He cares for humans in distinct and special ways. He cares for you and the way that you view your body. How would things be different if you saw your body through the eyes of your Creator: very good? After all, God found so much importance in the physical body that He gave Himself one through Jesus putting on flesh.[1]

Our Uniqueness

"I praise you for I am fearfully and wonderfully made.
Wonderful are your works; my soul knows it very well."
~ Psalm 139:14 (ESV)

PSALM 139:14 IS MORE about God than it is about ourselves, contrary to what it may seem like on first reading. David, the author, wrote this out of a heart posture of praise and gratitude for God's intentionality in His creation. Jesus proclaims in John 15:1 that He is *"the true vine, and [His] Father is the vinedresser."* A vinedresser is a person who prunes and cultivates or is a worker of the soil. A vinedresser must always be watchful, diligent, and meticulous in his work. It is beautiful, then, that Our Father is a vinedresser! If a vinedresser is like this with his vineyard, how much more is God watchful, diligent, and meticulous in His creation of us? We are God's masterpiece, after all (Ephesians 2:10).

We see God's intentional crafting of us in studying Exodus 25-30, the building and designing of the Tabernacle. The Tabernacle was a type of temple, a temporary dwelling place where Heaven and earth could meet. We see in these 5 chapters that God has a purpose for how He wanted the Tabernacle, and God also has complete sovereignty over all things. God gives intrinsic beauty to the place![2] After Jesus' death and resurrection, when God gave us the Holy Spirit, our bodies are now called temples of the Holy Spirit (1 Corinthians 6:19). God makes His dwelling place in us! Similarly, 1 Kings 6-8 is an extensive description of Soloman building the temple (specificity even down to the cubit!).

Therefore, knowing that God designs intentionally and cannot make mistakes, we are given the freedom to look at what others may depict as "flaws" of ourselves and turn it into thanksgiving. The phrase "body image disturbance" is typically more general and focuses more on body dissatisfaction around shape and size. Body dysmorphia is when there is an overemphasis on a specific body part.[3] A perceived imperfection about oneself can lead to intense emotional distress and a loss of a sense of presence in the day-to-day, or even a lost sense of identity. Have you noticed a tendency to only see your pimples when you look in the mirror? Do you only wear certain clothes to try to cover up scars? Do you edit your teeth in every picture? Are you constantly trying to flex to see your muscle tone? The Lord makes us unique for His glory! The texture of your hair, skin tone, birthmarks, scars, body size, etc., were chosen by God!

The world may counteract body dysmorphia by saying we need more self-love, and this is not entirely wrong. The second commandment says, "*Love your neighbor as yourself*" (Mark 12:31). Note: as yourself! Loving others can easily become a moral action driven by the desire to feel good about oneself or even appear in some way to others rather than from the overflow of a sincere heart saturated in God's love. In other words, loving others can easily be out of selfish ambition (Philippians 2:3), especially when you are not loving yourself. Nonetheless, we are called to love ourselves and others because "he first loved us" (1 John 4:19).[A]

Self-love and self-esteem are not synonymous. Merriam Webster defines self-love as "an appreciation of one's own worth or virtue," whereas self-esteem is defined as "confidence and satisfaction in oneself."[4,5] Another way to think about self-esteem is the opinion of yourself. With a biblical worldview, we know it is Christ who gives us our inherent worth and value as made in the image of God. Thus, the biblical commandment of self-love is marked with humility. On the other hand, self-esteem can easily be rooted in pride apart from God because we have no good apart from Him (Psalm 16:2, Mark 10:18). Tim Keller expounds on this with his claim in *The Freedom of Self-Forgetfulness* that "our only solution to low self-esteem is pride."[6] This is because self-esteem is focused on elevating the self above all and taking the focus off of God. Self-esteem assigns worth based on characteristics about yourself instead of your identity as a daughter or son of Jesus. It neglects the reality of the Imago Dei.

C.S. Lewis, in *Mere Christianity,* furthers this idea by stating, "It is competitiveness that is at the very heart of pride."[7] Ask yourself: are there subconscious competitions sliding into your thoughts like, "I eat more or less *than them,* I am more or less physically fit *than them,* etc.?" Note this "than them" mentality. Why does this happen? Anything that threatens your pride becomes a big deal. Therefore, if you have a season of high *body* self-esteem, there will inevitably be more anxiety about your body changing because you feel you need to maintain it. Likewise, if you have higher *body* self-esteem when your skin is super clear versus when those inevitable breakouts arise, you will be left in shambles. Extending love to yourself in the way Jesus extends love to you is how we can stop our ever-changing bodies from throwing us into chronic emotional roller coasters.ᴬ Once again, *"We love because He first loved us!"* (1 John 4:19). Through loving yourself as God loves you, self-esteem can then come to hold a proper position in our life: a means of confidence that is not shaken by what the world has to say about you because of the confidence you have in what God says about you.

· · ·

PRAYER

Dear God,

I praise You for making me both fearfully and wonderfully. You know me better than I know myself. I confess the ways that I have fallen into the trap of thinking of my body too much. Our bodies are good gifts that You gave us to live this life in. You are a good Father, and You did not make mistakes when you created me. Thank You for my body. Show me what it is like to see it as a gift from You.

In Jesus' name, Amen!

FOOTNOTES:

A. We acknowledge that self-love may be difficult or even impossible for some individuals struggling with depression or other mental health issues. If this is the case for you, please seek help from a counselor, preferably a biblical counselor.

SOURCES:

1. Allberry S. *What God Has to Say about Our Bodies: How the Gospel Is Good News for Our Physical Selves.* Crossway; August 3, 2021.

2. Gilbert R. *Image RESTored - Includes Six-Session Video Series.* David C Cook; 2023.

3. Understanding the difference between body dysmorphia, self-esteem, and negative body image. Discovery Mood & Anxiety Program. https://discoverymood.com/blog/understanding-difference-body-dysmorphia-self-esteem-negative-body-image/#:~:text=Body%20 dysmorphic%20disorder%20(BDD)%2C,to%20how%20peo ple%20see%20themselves. Published August 7, 2019. Accessed May 13, 2024.

4. "Self-love". Merriam-webster.com Dictionary, Merriam-Webster, https://www.merriam-webster.com/dictionary/self-love. Published 2020.

5. "Self-esteem". Merriam-webster.com Dictionary, Merriam-Webster, https://www.merriam-

webster.com/dictionary/self-esteem. Published 2019.

6. Keller TJ. *The Freedom of Self-Forgetfulness: The Path to True Christian Joy.* New York City, New York: 10 Publishing; March 27, 2012.

7. Lewis CS. *Mere Christianity.* HarperCollins Publishers; 1952.

16

RELATIONSHIPS

Attraction

"For the Lord does not see as man sees; for the man looks at the outward appearance, but the Lord looks at the heart."
~ 1 Samuel 16:7 (ESV)

THE IDEA OF physical attraction is one of the most prominent reasons why Western culture is so obsessed with body image. That is because this culture is infiltrated with things like pornography, romantic movies and novels, revealing models, social media content, and more. It is rare to get through a day without seeing an edited picture of someone's body, hearing something sexual in a song, or passing by an obscene billboard. These things that surround us create the idea that attraction is found in our outward physical appearance. However, when we meditate on the Lord's heart, 1 Samuel 16:7

challenges this thought. The Lord does not look at our physical appearance; He looks at our hearts.

God's Word should be the relational and directional basis for our lives. Proverbs 31:30 reminds us, "*Charm is deceitful, and beauty is vain, but a woman who fears the Lord is to be praised.*" When an individual fears the Lord, their entire life revolves around a reverence for God. When someone's life surrounds Christ, they become more like Christ. When someone becomes more like Christ, the fruits of the Spirit "*love, joy, peace, patience, kindness, goodness, faithfulness, gentleness, [and] self-control*" are more clearly expressed (Galatians 5:22). Likewise, when someone is more like Christ, what they are attracted to will thus become more like what Christ is attracted to: the heart! Physical appearance does not show someone's values, character, or faithfulness to God. It is okay to have preferences, and that may even be your initial motivation to approach someone. That being said, if you are focusing mainly on appearance instead of heart, (as we learned from Proverbs 31:30) you are seeking vain and deceitful things instead of pursuing someone who fears the Lord.

God is always more concerned with our heart's intentions than any outward image. 1 Peter 3:3-4 dives deeper into this, commanding women in the Roman upper-class society to "*not let the adorning be external- the braiding of your hair and the putting on of gold jewelry, or the clothing you wear- but let your adorning be the hidden person of the heart with the imperishable beauty of a gentle and quiet spirit, which in God's sight is very precious.*" This does not mean women should not get dressed up. It is a gift to get dressed up and feel beautiful! The point, however, is that your true beauty is found on the inside and is unchanged regardless of how you look and what you wear.

Some might respond, "Well, yes, God looks at the heart, but people don't; therefore, I need to be attractive to find a spouse." This is a very prevalent view in the Christian community. There are many people who know finding someone who values your heart is important but fall under the convincing thought that they need to lose weight to be "more attractive." It is easy to believe no one will recognize their heart unless they first are noticed by their external appearance. They use their external appearance as the hook to lure someone into their true self. Maybe you have heard it before that "the bait you lure them in with is the bait you are going to keep them with." If this bait was your body, you are in a tricky position, considering our bodies will forever be changing.

What happens when you have a baby, get wrinkles, grow gray hair, have a breakout, or get injured? If you do not want to be in this exhausting mindset forever trying to keep someone around with the way your body looks, take a broader view of attraction that views attraction in more ways than just physical appearance. In other words, look for someone pursuing the heart of Christ! Think of what your own definition of beauty is. Let the reality that you have been approved of by God take priority over the need to find approval in a potential mate. After all, are you thinking more about how you can invest in the Kingdom or more about how your body looks to others?

Singleness

"There is no fear in love, but perfect love casts out all fear."
~ 1 John 4:18 (ESV)

WHETHER OR NOT we get married, we were made for relationships. We see this perfectly in the Triune God! As fallen humans, we want other people to satisfy our desire for connection and belonging and, therefore, make us feel secure. It is not a bad thing to desire connection, but the problem arises when we *use* people to resolve our insecurities because people are imperfect and will always disappoint. When we look beneath our insecurities, we often find fear. This could be a fear of being rejected, being alone forever, or being a second choice. More than likely, though, there will be one insecurity or another, whether it is around body image, personality, charisma, you name it!

Dating someone to resolve personal insecurities is not only using that person, but it may also be feeding into your unhealthy behavior. In other words, if you are regularly engaging in disordered eating patterns and then get noticed by the opposite sex, it is easy to think, "I had to do this to get noticed, so I have to do this to continue getting noticed." If other people and circumstances determine our contentment levels, we will constantly seek change when we lose that contentment (even if temporarily). Sam Allberry, in his book *7 Myths of Singleness,* said, "When Jesus says He's the bread of life, He's saying that He's to our soul what bread is to the stomach."[1] Like food is a necessary component of survival for our physical bodies, Christ is a necessary component of survival for our spiritual selves. Just like we cannot replace supplements for food to survive, we cannot put people in the place of God (the one who is supposed to reign in our lives) and expect ever to be satisfied or truly alive.

No person is complete by himself because He was made for a relationship with God and others. This is another example of how humans are made to reflect God. Even Jesus, being fully God and fully man, is in a Triune relationship: God the Father, Son, and Holy Spirit! The Scriptures claim, "It is not good for man to be alone," but this does not refer to singleness being bad (Genesis 2:18). In fact, in 1 Corinthians 7, Paul writes about singleness in a favorable light. Why? Allbery explains how "singleness gives [him] the capacity for a range of friendships [he] otherwise wouldn't be able to sustain if [he] was married." [1] It also gives you more capacity to serve the church and love your community around you sacrificially. Singleness shows the sufficiency of the gospel, while marriage displays the image of the gospel.[1]

In Heaven, there is only one marriage: Christ and His church fully restored. Therefore, Genesis 2:18 means that it is not good for us to live in isolation. You do not have to be married or have a romantic partner to be in community with others. You can be single and live a very fulfilling and gospel-centered life!

Both singleness and marriage bring about gifts and challenges.

However, culture (and the church!) overprioritizes being in a romantic relationship and sees singleness as a gift to give away. It is tempting to think of gifts in terms of individual fulfillment, but perfect fulfillment is found in Christ alone.[1] God's Word challenges us to think of our uniquely given gifts for building up the church. After all, what is our purpose here on earth? Acts 20:24 reads: "*But I do not account my life of any value nor as precious to myself, if only I may finish my course and the ministry that I received from the Lord Jesus, to testify to the gospel of the grace of God.*" This is a life motto we should adopt for our purpose here on earth, and this has nothing to do with whether you are single or married!

Singleness is not an inferior state, and short-term or long-term singleness is not an issue with your body. Still, this can be a tempting thought when you are not feeding your soul rightly. Proverbs 4:23 says, "*Above all else, guard your heart, for it is the wellspring of life.*" When we feel these lies rising, we must "*take captive every thought to make it obedient to Christ*" (2 Corinthians 10:5). What you give attention to is where your devotion starts. What are you more attentive to: His word or "What I Eat in a Day" videos, the family of God (community) or reality TV shows, prayer, or social media stalking? God is most glorified in us when we are most satisfied in Him.[2] Relationships with people will not satisfy.

Despite what people may think, marriage does not guarantee perfect companionship or the repair of any body image struggles. There are many married people who feel very lonely and insecure in their marriage. Likewise, there are many single people who have incredibly deep, intimate relationships in their lives! The *only* guarantee of complete, consistent, fulfilling companionship we have for life is Christ because when we have chosen to believe in Him, we are indwelt by the Holy Spirit (Romans 8:10). God tells us he will never leave nor forsake us (Deuteronomy 31:8)!

Marriage

"Wives, submit to your own husbands, as to the Lord...
Husbands, love your wives, as Christ loved the church and gave
himself up for her."
~ Ephesians 5:22, 25 (ESV)

MARRIAGE IS ANOTHER reflection of the gospel, yet it is imperfect because of the ways that we, as humans, carry it out. The purpose of marriage is to point us to Christ. Wives are to submit to their husbands, as we all are to submit to the leadership and authority of Christ in our lives. Husbands are to love their wives and lay down their lives for them as Christ loves the Church and sacrificed Himself for her. Living as a woman in the twenty-first century, a time that values women more than any previous generation, it can be hard to grasp the idea of giving up freedom as women to submit to our husbands. As men, it can feel intimidating to love your wife and lay down your life, your desires, and your dreams for her. Contrary to popular belief, though, submission is actually a gift, just as husbands loving their wives is a gift. Both sides have an active role. It is easy to see submission as restraining, but when a husband lays down his life for his wife, submission is seen in a different light. After all, submission mirrors Christ's submission to the Father (1 Corinthians 11:13, Hebrews 10:7, John 4:34, John 8:28).[3] Submission and the meaning of marriage are excellent topics to study, but for now, let's turn our focus to how marriage relates to our struggles with food and body image.[A]

Being married is not "better" than being single. As mentioned earlier in this chapter, the Apostle Paul would say that singleness is a greater calling and it is *"better to be single"* (1 Corinthians 7:8). Both Biblical and modern societies alike place a high value on marriage and a very low value on singleness, which is directly contradictory to Paul's teachings. Because of this, many women (and men) believe that marriage is the ultimate calling in their lives, and once they get married, they will have all of the validation they need around their bodies and will no longer have any reason to be insecure. This could not be further from the truth. While a loving and Godly husband should respect his wife's body by speaking positively about it, having validation from a man does not "fix" negative body thoughts. This is also true for men. A Godly wife should also respect her husband's body in the same way. Negative body image has nothing to do with what our bodies actually look like and everything to do with our insecurities about ourselves.

Take, for example, my client Shelby.[B] When Shelby started working with me (Anna Marie), she had been married for about 8 years. In those years, she gave birth to two wonderful children. She came to me because she initially wanted to work on "losing the baby weight." I was very transparent with her upfront, saying that I take a non-diet approach and that weight loss would not be our goal. She decided she still wanted to meet with me and try something new. At our first appointment, she shared that her husband was pressuring her to change her body and "go back to the body he married." He shared with her that he was no longer attracted to her postpartum body. She was feeling the pressure to try to look the same way she did on her wedding day. On her wedding day, she was in the depths of a life-threatening eating disorder, and the only thing she could remember about that day was how hungry she was. This is all too common! Diet culture is the loudest around wedding planning and postpartum. Shelby's husband was feeding into the diet culture narrative that bodies should never change, and we should spend all of our time and energy attempting to shrink them. What both Shelby and her husband were failing to understand was that attraction is more than just physical. The problem here was not only believing that different body shapes and sizes are better than others, but it was also a deeper heart issue. Shelby's husband was living in the sin of seeing his attraction to his wife as nothing more than her body, and Shelby was in the sin of idolizing her former body and not practicing gratitude toward her current body. Both of these sinful struggles led to disunity in their marriage, and until they let the Lord into this and confessed and repented, they were unable to see meaningful changes.

In an ideal world, all married women would have husbands who love their bodies and speak about them like Solomon describes his wife in the book of Song of Solomon (or Song of Songs, depending on your translation). However, the difficult reality is that we all live in a diet culture, and many husbands "encourage" their wives to pursue body changes. In the same way, many women may also push their husbands to "not get a dad bod" or to try to manipulate their bodies as well. In the garden of Eden, before sin entered the world, Adam and Eve were naked together *"and not ashamed"* (Genesis 2:25).

Humans being ashamed of our bodies is a product of the fall and sin. There is a value to modesty and covering yourself in front of others, but in the context of marriage, we were designed to be naked with each other and unashamed.

The sexual revolution was a movement that started in the 1960s, along with the feminist movement. The birth control pill was invented, and women could enjoy sex without the possibility of an unplanned pregnancy.[4] This led to a major increase in women engaging in premarital sex and a decrease in social stigma around this. In response to this, the Church began the purity movement in the 80's and 90's. The main message of the purity movement was to encourage everyone to "save sex for marriage," which is a good and Godly message, except that it also emphasized unhelpful, shame-based tactics mostly aimed at women.[5] These focused on women "not causing their brother to stumble," which places a high amount of blame and responsibility on women.[5] The culture was pushing one thing (sexual "freedom" outside of marriage), and the Church was pushing the opposite (keeping yourself pure for marriage). There is a major problem with both of these movements: the self, not Christ, is at the center.

While saving sex for marriage is good and right, it is not solely the woman's responsibility. The responsibility is on both believers, and a woman (or man) is not "impure" if she (or he) stumbles before marriage. This relates to body image because our past and present sins can lead to us feeling worse about our bodies (feeling "impure" or like "damaged goods"), which robs us from enjoying a good thing in marriage.

God created sex, after all, to be enjoyed within the covenant of marriage. Sex outside of marriage, however, is sinful, and like any other sin, it should be avoided (Hebrews 13:4, 1 Corinthians 6:18). If you have found yourself in the sin of engaging in sexual acts outside of marriage, there is grace for that, too! Jesus died for all of our sins. Purity culture in the church fuels shame around sins that are fully forgiven and covered by the blood of Christ. If reading this stirs up shame, remember that Jesus' sacrifice was enough to forgive every single one of your sins. We should, however, strive to turn away from our sexual sin in the present and future. Romans 6:1-2 reminds us that we should not continue to sin so that grace may abound. We have died to our sins, and we can praise God that we do not have to live in bondage to them anymore!

In marriage, sexual intimacy is designed to be a physical expression of Christ's covenant love.[6] It can be extremely difficult to enjoy sex in the context of marriage if you are consumed with thoughts about your body and how you look. Ephesians 5:31-32 discusses how, in marriage, a husband and wife become one flesh. Therefore, our bodies belong to our spouse, as they belong to the Lord (1 Corinthians 7:1-5). Scripture does not discuss our bodies looking a certain way in the context of intimacy. Letting negative body thoughts get in the way of having pleasurable and frequent sex with your spouse is another way that the enemy tries to rob us of the joy that is only found in walking with Christ.

While marriage and oneness with a spouse are good gifts, marriage is not the "fix" for all of your body image struggles. Putting that pressure on a spouse will remove the joy of intimacy with a partner. God wants us to be free from negative body image. A spouse is not the key to freedom; only Jesus is!

. . .

PRAYER

Dear God,

Thank You for the way that You created us. You are a good Creator and Father, and You do not make mistakes. You have given your creation the gift of attraction. You look deeper beyond the physical appearance and see the heart. Show me what it looks like to become more like You in how I view others. Help me to see the good gift of where You have me in this moment, and help me to lean on my community so that I am not living life alone. You love to give good gifts, so I thank You for the gifts you have provided for me in this season.

In Jesus' name, Amen.

FOOTNOTE:

A. A great biblical resource on marriage is *The Meaning of Marriage* by Timothy and Kathy Keller.

B. For the purposes of this book and maintaining confidentiality, the names used in the examples have all been changed.

SOURCES:

1. Allberry S. *7 Myths about Singleness*. Crossway; February 28, 2019.

2. Piper J. *Desiring God: Meditations of a Christian Hedonist*. Portland, Oregon: Multnomah Books; 1986.

3. Keller K. *The Meaning of Marriage: Facing the Complexities of Commitment with the Wisdom of God*. Penguin Books; November 5, 2013.

4. PBS. The Pill and the Sexual Revolution | American Experience | PBS. Pbs.org. Published 2019. https://www.pbs.org/wgbh/americanexperience/features/pill-and-sexual-revolution/

5. Slattery, J. Purity Culture: Lose the Lies, Keep Your Faith - Authentic Intimacy. https://www.authenticintimacy.com/purity-culture-lose-the-lies-keep-your-faith/. Published February 26, 2021. Accessed June 20, 2024.

6. Slattery J. How to say "Yes, Yes, Yes!" after "No, No, No!" - Authentic Intimacy. https://www.authenticintimacy.com/how-to-say-yes-yes-yes-after-no-no-no/. Published May 9, 2016. Accessed June 20, 2024.

17

MOVEMENT

Movement Defined

"For while bodily training is of some value, godliness is of value in every way, as it holds promise for the present life and also for the life to come."
~ 1 Timothy 4:8 (ESV)

WHEN PEOPLE HAVE a disordered relationship with their food and body, there is often a disordered relationship around exercise, too. Exercise can then be used as another tool to manipulate your body shape and size and compensate for food intake. However, just as one can have food freedom, one can have exercise freedom! Like the ever-changing "beauty" trends, fitness trends are also forever changing. Sometimes, it is "cool" to be training for the next half or full marathon, while at other times, it is pilates reformer, then boot camp and high-intensity interval training (HIIT), then strength training, and so on. At the root of this, there are no black-and-white rules to the "right way" to move your body! Just like finding balance in the food you eat is important, finding balance in exercise is equally important. Our bodies do need movement, but too much will lead to our detriment. You can have too much of any good thing. Even scripture shows us that physical training is only of *"some value"* (1 Timothy 4:8). Living a life of godliness is of much more importance than our levels of training here on earth.

Your body needs food for movement. Period. Your body uses macronutrients (carb, protein, fat) for fuel during exercise. To sustain a workout, minimize muscle fatigue, and maintain blood sugar levels during exercise, glycogen (the storage form of glucose from carbs) is needed! Hence, consuming more carbohydrates will extend your endurance. Additionally, to promote muscle growth and maintain proper repair and recovery, protein is needed! When performing an exercise, your muscle fibers undergo microtears, and without proper energy intake, they will not be able to rebuild.

Aerobic and anaerobic exercise are the two most commonly heard terms when it comes to working out. Essentially, aerobic exercise is a form of movement where the oxygen demands of your body can be met. This involves movement that is lower in intensity because it requires longer endurance (distance running or walking, swimming, cycling, Zumba/dancing, yoga/barre/pilates, etc.). Do not overlook stretching and mobility as forms of exercise, too. The initial source of fuel for the aerobic system is muscle glycogen. The other fuel sources (and main fuel source) for the aerobic system are triglycerides in your cells and free fatty acids in the blood. Once again, fat and carbs are needed for this. Insufficient and inconsistent energy intake will thus hinder your body's ability to get the required fuel it needs to sustain exercise.

Anaerobic exercise, on the other hand, is a form of movement where your body cannot keep up with the oxygen needed due to the higher intensity and shorter duration (sprinting, weightlifting, HIIT, plyometric training, etc.). Blood glucose is the main fuel source used in the anaerobic system. Therefore, if you have insufficient and inconsistent carbohydrate intake, your muscles will have inadequate muscle glycogen stores for both initiation of aerobic exercise and maintenance of anaerobic exercise. Muscle fatigue occurs when the glucose supply is inadequate.

Another factor in aerobic and anaerobic exercise is the type of muscle fibers used. The predominant muscle fiber in aerobic exercise is Type 1 (otherwise known as "slow twitch"). On the other hand, the predominant muscle fiber in anaerobic exercise is Type 2 (otherwise known as "fast twitch"). The proportion of muscle fiber types in our bodies is genetically determined. Therefore, if you notice you enjoy particular forms of exercise more than others, that is likely for a biological reason! Take two people: one genuinely enjoys longer-distance walking or running, and the other genuinely enjoys strength training. The one who enjoys longer-distance walking or running may very well have more Type 1 muscle fibers, whereas the one who enjoys strength may have more Type 2 muscle fibers. This means that you do not have to force yourself to like a certain form of movement or "get better at it" just because other people enjoy it. It may not be joyful for you, but that is okay. The forms of movement that feel joyful to you may not be joyful to others.

It is also important to acknowledge that for some people, movement in general is just not enjoyable. A small percentage of the population are actually "exercise non-responders."[1] These individuals have either no response or a negative response to specific exercise regimens.[2] These people have a very low amount of both Type 1 and Type 2 muscle fibers. These individuals can exercise, but no amount or type of exercise will give them the endorphins that most individuals get from their preferred form of movement. Improving sleep hygiene and removing emotional stressors can help with exercise non-responsiveness, but for these individuals, exercise is simply more difficult.[1] If this is you, remember that God made you with intentionality, and this is no mistake. There is no need to "white knuckle" or force yourself to repeatedly do an activity that feels like a chore. For these individuals, as well as for everyone else, we actually get movement through non-exercise activity thermogenesis (or NEAT). NEAT is any non-planned form of exercise. This includes things like fidgeting, walking in the parking lot from your car, cooking, cleaning, and taking stairs, to name a few. The point is that you are moving your body throughout the day in ways you may not even realize!

Movement provides many benefits that have nothing to do with weight or physique, and movement is so much more than even the physical benefits. Movement can be a way to connect with God. Walking, running, hiking, swimming, climbing, and biking (etc.) gets you into the outdoors to enjoy God's creation! You can listen to the birds chirping and sounds of laughter. You can feel wind, water, and sunlight hit your skin. You can also bring friends into this to enjoy the presence of community. Community can be enjoyed indoors, too, by taking a class or lifting weights with a friend. 1 Timothy 6:17 exhorts us to truly enjoy all that God has given us in this life!

Our bodies carry us through so much every day. Life is a marathon, not a sprint. We are in it for the long haul (as long as the Lord gives us breath in our lungs), so it is crucial to take care of our bodies. Ultimately, it's important to find what is maintainable for you. Going to the gym six to seven times a week, working out more than once a day, and repeatedly doing high-intensity days back to back is not going to be maintainable for very long. This all-or-nothing mentality leads to burnout from exercise and not wanting to do it anymore. No matter how much we try, our outer selves will slowly decay (2 Corinthians 4:16), yet Christ will transform them (Philippians 3:20-21). If you are able, the next time you exercise, give thanks to God because not everyone has this ability in our broken world. Pursuing body change through exercise is vanity (Ecclesiastes 1), but joy is found in receiving exercise with thanksgiving (1 Timothy 4:4).

God Does not Value Being Active in the Same Way We Do

"...and the lame I will make the remnant, and those who were cast off, a strong nation; and the Lord will reign over them in Mount Zion from this time forth and forevermore."
~ Micah 4:7 (ESV)

IN DISCUSSING MOVEMENT, it is important to keep in mind that some people physically cannot move. People in early eating disorder recovery, or recovery from any other physical ailments such as early cancer, a stroke, or post-operative procedures are unable to move their bodies for a certain amount of time. Movement in these individuals would do more harm than good. Just like in the Bible, some people are paralyzed from accidents or unable to walk from birth. The Bible refers to these individuals as being "lame." This is not a bad or a mocking term; it is simply an adjective. God values all of His image bearers, not just those who are able-bodied. If God did not value individuals with physical disabilities, he would not include them in scripture.

Take Mephibosheth, Jonathan's son, as an example. When Mephibosheth was 5 years old, he fell and became "lame" (2 Samuel 4:4). Jonathan feared the Lord and gave us an example of what Christ-centered friendship should look like. In 1 Samuel 19, Jonathan is good friends with David and protects him from Saul, Jonathan's father, who seeks to kill David. Observing the life of David, it is obvious that his friendship with Jonathan was important and cherished. At the beginning of David's reign as king, he had several military victories, and then he appointed his royal officials. David then asked if there was anyone else from Saul's line that he could show kindness to for the sake of his friend Jonathan (2 Samuel 9:1). Thus, in 2 Samuel 9, David showed extreme kindness to Mephibosheth, even though Mephibosheth did nothing to earn David's affection. David did not see Mephibosheth as "less than" because of his disability. David cared about who he was, not what he did or did not do. David was an imperfect, sinful man, but he was a man after God's own heart (1 Samuel 13:14, Acts 13:22). David was a foreshadowing of Jesus, the perfect and better King who was to come.

In the same way that David loved Mephibosheth because of *who* he was, the Lord loves us because we are His, and He calls us to Himself. He does not value movement or being able-bodied the way that we do. When you feel guilty for skipping a workout or for not moving your body in the way that you feel that you "should," remember that this is not sinful, and that guilt has no place when it comes to deciding to move or not move your body.

This is not to say never engage in movement if you are able to, as there are both physical and mental health benefits of moving your body. This includes things like regulation of circadian rhythm, improving your cardiovascular system, and pumping endorphins. Studies show that 12 minutes of lower-intensity exercise can reduce impulsivity, improve mood, and help with sleep.[3] There are benefits to moving, but there are also benefits to resting. And remember, for those in eating disorder recovery, stopping exercise may actually be more beneficial (and may be needed) for you physically and mentally. In this case, it is vital to talk with your treatment team about the best course of action.

Whether you choose to move your body is up to you, but there is no moral value to this decision. We can see from the example of David and Mephibosheth that it is far more important that your identity is secure in belonging to the King. When we rightly see that this is more important, we can put movement in its right place - a good thing, but not an ultimate thing.

. . .

PRAYER

Dear God,

Thank You for calling me Yours. You are such a good God. I praise You for the way that You created me. Help me to fight off guilty thoughts around moving or not moving. Remind me that my identity is secure in You, first and foremost. Show me what it looks like to honor You with the ways that I move my body and rest.

In Jesus' name, amen.

S O U R C E S :

1. Pickering C, Kiely J. Do non-responders to exercise exist—
    and if so, what should we do about them? *Sports Medicine.*
    2018;49(1):1-7. doi:https://doi.org/10.1007/s40279-018-
    01041-1
2. Bouchard C, Rankinen T. Individual differences in response
    to regular physical activity. *Medicine and Science in Sports
    and Exercise.* 2001;33(Supplement):S446-S451.
    doi:https://doi.org/10.1097/00005768-200106001-00013
3. Mahindru A, Patil P, Agrawal V. Role of physical activity on
    mental health and well-being: A review. *Cureus.* 2023;15(1).
    doi:https://doi.org/10.7759/cureus.33475

18

SUPPORTING SOMEONE WITH AN EATING DISORDER

*"This is my commandment, that you love one another
as I have loved you."*
~ John 15:12 (ESV)

IF YOU PICKED up this book to gain practical tools for how to support a loved one with an eating disorder, we hope you have gained some insight and seen the importance of letting the Lord in. Whether you are reading this for yourself or for a friend, child, spouse, or family member, the best place to begin supporting that loved one is to pray for them. Ephesians 6:18 reminds us to pray at all times for the Lord's people. Even if your loved one is not ready to open up to you about their struggles, the power of prayer is the most helpful tool you can use. Pray for courage to confess, confidence to face recovery head-on, and the community to surround them with encouragement. Eating disorders (like any sin) thrive in isolation. The eating disorder wants your loved one to believe that it is "not that bad" and that they can "recover on their own." This could not be further from the truth.

As mentioned throughout this book, living in a community with other followers of Jesus is so important. If you are reading this, it is clear that you care deeply about your loved one who is struggling, and praise God, this person has you! Being present is the second most important thing you can do to support someone struggling. To simply be there with a person suffering in solidarity toward a mutual goal of healing has great value. 1 Thessalonians 5:11 speaks hopefully about the Day of the Lord to come and tells us in the meantime to encourage one another and lift each other up. If you are reading this book to support someone in recovery, be encouraged that you are walking this out!

It can be tempting when our loved one tells us about their food and body struggles to try to "fix" the problem. After all, when they complain about disliking their body, it is easy to give them affirmations and disagree with their assessment. For example, when a loved one says, "I feel fat," and you respond by saying, "You're not fat, you're beautiful," this is seldom helpful. Not only will your loved one continue to ask for reassurance that they are not fat (or any perceived negative adjective about their body), but the response of "you're not fat, you're beautiful" implies that fat is the opposite of beautiful and validates the fears that the eating disorder is telling them. Remember, fat is not a bad thing; it is simply an adjective. Fat is also not a feeling. Assuring and reassuring them that what the eating disorder says is not true does not support them in recovery. Instead, being a listening ear over offering a solution can be more helpful. An example of a different response in the previous scenario could be responding with, "I am really sorry that you are feeling that way. Please, tell me more about what that means for you." This response opens the door for your loved one to slowly peel back layers and tell you more about what is actually going on. Asking open-ended questions (not yes or no questions) is key. Often, when your loved one is using adjectives (such as fat, ugly, unattractive, big, etc.) to describe feelings, there is a deeper emotion (such as fear, worry, anger, etc.) that they want to discuss with you, but they do not know how to describe it. We see a biblical command against trying to "fix" in James 1:19, which says, *"be quick to hear and slow to speak,"* granted this is often easier said than done.

Supporting someone with an eating disorder can be extremely difficult. If you are a caregiver of someone with an eating disorder, getting your own support from the local church or Biblical counselor can make a big difference. Philippians 2:4 does command you to put your loved one's needs before your own; however, it does not command neglecting yourself. In fact, neglecting care for yourself can lead to the detriment of both of you.

In conclusion, four practical ways you can support someone with an eating disorder are to pray for them, be present with them and spend quality time in the community with them, listen more than you speak, and get your own support if needed. We were not created to do recovery alone, so your support of them is important.

PRAYER

Dear God,

I pray for my loved one in recovery. You know their story, and You walk alongside them. Please walk alongside me and help me to offer a listening ear to them. I care so deeply for their heart, and I know You do too. Recovery is so hard, so I ask You to be with them and meet them where they are today. Be with me as I support and love them. Help me to show them more of You.

In Jesus' name, amen.

CONCLUSION

"Walk in a manner worthy of the calling to which
you have been called."
~ Ephesians 4:1b (ESV)

YOU'VE MADE IT to the end, so congratulations! As you learned about being made in the image of God, it is our hope that you challenged your beliefs about food and body through the lens of the gospel. We barely touched on the topics of food and nutrition in the first five chapters for a reason: it is more important that you know God's character than for you to read a book about nutrition. While nutrition is our passion, nothing compares to truly knowing Christ Jesus as Lord and Savior (Philippians 3:8). Understanding basic nutrition is great, but we must see nutrition (as well as every topic) through the lens of the gospel. True freedom is found when you begin to view the world through God's Word. Adopting this view of the world is important because Scripture is without error and is the only path to joy on this side of heaven.

The second half of this book covered hot topics in the Church, where diet culture frequently shows up. We learned about gluttony, fasting, feasting, self-control, body image, attraction, and movement. If any of these topics were difficult to read, we encourage you to meditate on the scriptures that were mentioned throughout the chapters and ask God for wisdom and understanding. If you are still struggling to grasp these topics, consider seeking professional help from a Biblical counselor or Registered Dietitian.

Full freedom from food and body struggles is possible with the help of the Holy Spirit. He wants to meet you in your struggles and walk with you day-by-day. If you only take one thing away from this book, we hope you learn that prayer is a powerful tool. While you can continue to learn about nutrition, science, and God's Word, the most powerful thing you can do is communicate with the Lord through prayer. Pray without ceasing to renew your mind daily (1 Thessalonians 5:17, Romans 12:2). You may disagree with us on our interpretation of scripture, and that is okay. Ultimately, our hope is that from reading this book, you have grown closer to the Lord. True freedom is found only in Jesus, and the Lord will sustain you, wherever you are on your journey (Numbers 6:24). Thank you for letting us into your story.

Hungry for more? Anna Marie and Stephanie have put together two free printable resources: A 6-week study guide and leader guide, so you can go through Nourished by Faith on your own or as part of a group.

Literarycanvas.com/nourished-by-faith-resources

ACKNOWLEDGEMENTS

We want to thank our beta readers: Brittani Oglesbee, Charity Wottrich, Calvin Burns, Liberty Davidson, Christopher Long, and Faith Crenshaw. Your feedback was invaluable and helped us make this book possible. We knew we could trust all of you with the task of reading through this book and making sure we were, first and foremost, rooting everything in the gospel and our hope that is only found in Jesus Christ.

We were intentional about who we asked to read and edit our book, choosing friends with degrees in writing, a Biblical counselor, a published author, and a church staff member. You all went above and beyond our expectations and made us think about our goals and intentions as we made our final edits in the book. We would also like to thank our friends and communities of believers around both of us for your unconditional support of us in writing this book.

As we mentioned countless times throughout the book, community is so important, so having the support of friends who love Jesus and love us has not only shown us more of Christ's character, but also helped us to persevere in completing this book. Lastly, we want to thank you, our readers, for reading our book and trusting us with your time as you read.